The ACT Toolbox for Kids

Acceptance & Commitment Therapy

170+ Activities and Games to Address Anxiety, Stress, Trauma, Motivation, Attachment, Self-Esteem, Distractibility, Depression, Behavioral Challenges, and More

Matt Ercolani, MS, LPC, NCC & Emily Heydt, PsyD

THE ACT (ACCEPTANCE AND COMMITMENT THERAPY) TOOLBOX FOR KIDS

Published by
PESI Publishing, Inc.
3839 White Ave
Eau Claire, WI 54703

Cover design by Emily Dyer
Interior design by Abby Isackson
Editing by Jenessa Jackson, PhD

ISBN 9781683739425 (paperback)
ISBN 9781683739784 (spiral bound)
ISBN 9781683739432 (ePUB)
ISBN 9781683739449 (ePDF)

Printed in the United States of America.

PESI Publishing
pesipublishing.com

Table of Contents

Introduction

Hey there!

We're so glad you picked up this book. Really.

Because if you're here, we're guessing you work with kids or teens—or the grown-ups who love them. And maybe, just maybe, you've had those moments in session where you think:

What do I do with this?

Why is this kid shutting down?

I've tried everything. Nothing's sticking.

We've been there. Many times.

This book was born out of those moments: the stuck ones, the tricky ones, the "how-do-I-reach-them?" ones. And if you've found yourself in that space (or anticipate that it's coming), you're in the right place.

We're here to offer something that has changed the way we do therapy: acceptance and commitment therapy, or ACT for short.

We'll be honest: One of us (Matt) was not immediately sold. At first glance, ACT sounded like a mash-up of buzzwords (mindfulness, defusion, etc.) all wrapped up in a quirky hexagon. But the more we used it, the more we saw real change. Not just symptom checklists going down, but actual, meaningful change in how kids related to their thoughts, emotions, and values—and how they *acted* on those values.

ACT became the framework we didn't know we were missing.

We wrote this workbook so that you wouldn't have to piece it together the long way. Whether you're a therapist, school psychologist, counselor, other helping professional, or just starting your helping journey in grad school, our hope is that this book will become your go-to shelf buddy, a hands-on, zero-fluff resource full of creative, developmentally appropriate ways to bring ACT to life in your sessions.

So . . . what even is ACT?

ACT (pronounced like the word *act*) is a therapy model that helps people live more meaningful, values-driven lives, regardless of tough thoughts, feelings, and circumstances. Instead of fighting against pain or trying to control every emotion, ACT teaches us to make space for it, respond with flexibility, and move toward what matters.

ACT is built around six core processes, often visualized as a hexagon (and affectionately called the hexaflex). They are:

- **Acceptance:** Making space for feelings, even the hard ones
- **Cognitive defusion:** Noticing thoughts without getting tangled up in them
- **Being present and mindful:** Contact with the present moment, showing up, here and now
- **Self-as-context:** Understanding that we are more than our thoughts, feelings, or roles
- **Values:** Clarifying what is most important
- **Committed action:** Taking steps toward those values, even when it's hard

ACT isn't about chasing happiness. It's about building psychological flexibility so that no matter what shows up, we can keep moving in the direction of our goals and values.

And because ACT isn't just a theory, this workbook is packed with kid-friendly worksheets, activities, metaphors, and games to help bring ACT off the page and into the therapy room. From pirate-themed values maps to pop-up blocker thought defusion tools, we've designed these resources to be playful, insightful, and ready to use.

This book is divided into six sections, each one centered around a core process from the ACT hexaflex. Within each section, you'll find a consistent four-part structure designed to help both you and your clients understand, practice, and apply each area of the hexaflex:

1. **Foundations and psychoeducation:** Kids tend to get the most out of skills when they understand the "why" behind them. In this section, we introduce the core ideas behind each ACT process in a way that is clear, relatable, and playful.
2. **Skill practice and application:** This section provides fun, hands-on activities that give kids an opportunity to try out each component of the hexaflex in concrete ways. Here, the concepts move from ideas on the page to lived skills that kids can carry into school, home, and daily life.
3. **Living through metaphor:** Metaphors bring the core process to life in vivid, relatable ways. By engaging with imagery, stories, and playful examples, kids learn how to notice, name, and work with their experiences without getting stuck in them.
4. **Mindfulness:** Mindfulness exercises help kids tune into the present moment with curiosity and kindness. This section provides playful, engaging ways to notice thoughts and feelings, make space for them, and respond with awareness rather than reactivity.

You can read it cover to cover if that's your style, but honestly, we built this to be a book you can flip through, dog-ear, and make your own. You know those beautiful books that sit untouched on your shelf, looking pretty but never really getting used? This isn't that book. We want you to use it. Jump to the section you need. Skip around. Scribble in the margins. More than anything, let it work for you and your clients.

One more thing . . .

This work isn't easy. Therapy (and especially therapy with kids) never is. You're balancing developmental needs, family dynamics, school stressors, diagnoses, and big emotions, all while trying to connect in a way that feels real and safe.

But you're not alone. We've built this book with you in mind, from our own messy, joyful, trial-and-error experiences in session. Our goal isn't perfection; it's connection. It's about giving kids the tools to navigate their internal world with curiosity, self-compassion, and courage.

So take a breath. Flip the page. Let's dive in.

It's time to ACT!

SECTION 1

Acceptance

In ACT, acceptance means learning to make space for all of our thoughts, feelings, and body sensations, even the tricky, uncomfortable, or painful ones. It doesn't mean we *like* those feelings or even *want* them around all the time. It also doesn't mean that we are accepting that *it is okay* that they are there. It simply means we stop spending our energy trying to push them away or pretend they don't exist, and accept that they are present.

Why accept the existence of unpleasant or unhelpful thoughts, feelings, and body sensations? Accepting sounds like giving up! In reality, that could not be further from the truth. Accepting means that we acknowledge the truth of the situation so that instead of wasting time trying to fight against reality, we can focus on *working with* reality as it is. There are certain circumstances that we cannot change and certain thoughts or feelings that we cannot fully avoid, and that is okay. Acceptance is about meeting life on life's terms so that we can move forward on our terms.

As a clinician, you might find yourself wondering how to explain acceptance to kids and caregivers without sounding like you are implying that we just need to "deal with it." In fact, the "just deal with it" idea is an excellent place to start when explaining what acceptance is *not*. When we tell ourselves to "just deal with it," there is an undercurrent of pushing down or ignoring our circumstances—without ever really dealing with "it" in the first place. Acceptance helps us put a name to the "it" and learn to let it visit us, but not take over.

Electric Jello

Therapeutic Rationale

The human brain is often compared to a computer, but imagine if that computer were made of jello with electricity running through it. Would you trust the informational output of a bowl of jello hooked up to a car battery? Of course not! And yet we treat the informational output of *our* electric jello (i.e., our thoughts and feelings) as fact. This activity introduces kids to the idea that their thoughts and feelings, while important, are not always accurate reflections of reality.

Goals

- Practice intellectual acceptance by observing thoughts and feelings without judgment
- Introduce a shared metaphor ("electric jello") that can be referred to throughout therapy

Materials

- *Electric Jello* template
- Writing utensil
- Crayons, markers, or colored pencils

Instructions

1. Introduce the concept of electric jello, gently poking fun at the absurdity of the idea.
2. Ask the client, "If you were taking a math test, would you rather have a calculator or a bowl of jello with a car battery hooked up to it? Why?" Use this to highlight how unreliable our brain's output can sometimes be.
3. Prompt the client to explore different thoughts or feelings that have caused them distress; have them write these down inside the bowl on the *Electric Jello* template.
4. Once the illustration is complete (and colored in as they desire), ask, "What do you notice about your own electric jello?" Use their answer to process the idea that thoughts are just thoughts, and feelings are just feelings.
5. Brainstorm strategies with the client to help them remember and apply the concept of electric jello moving forward.

Electric Jello Template

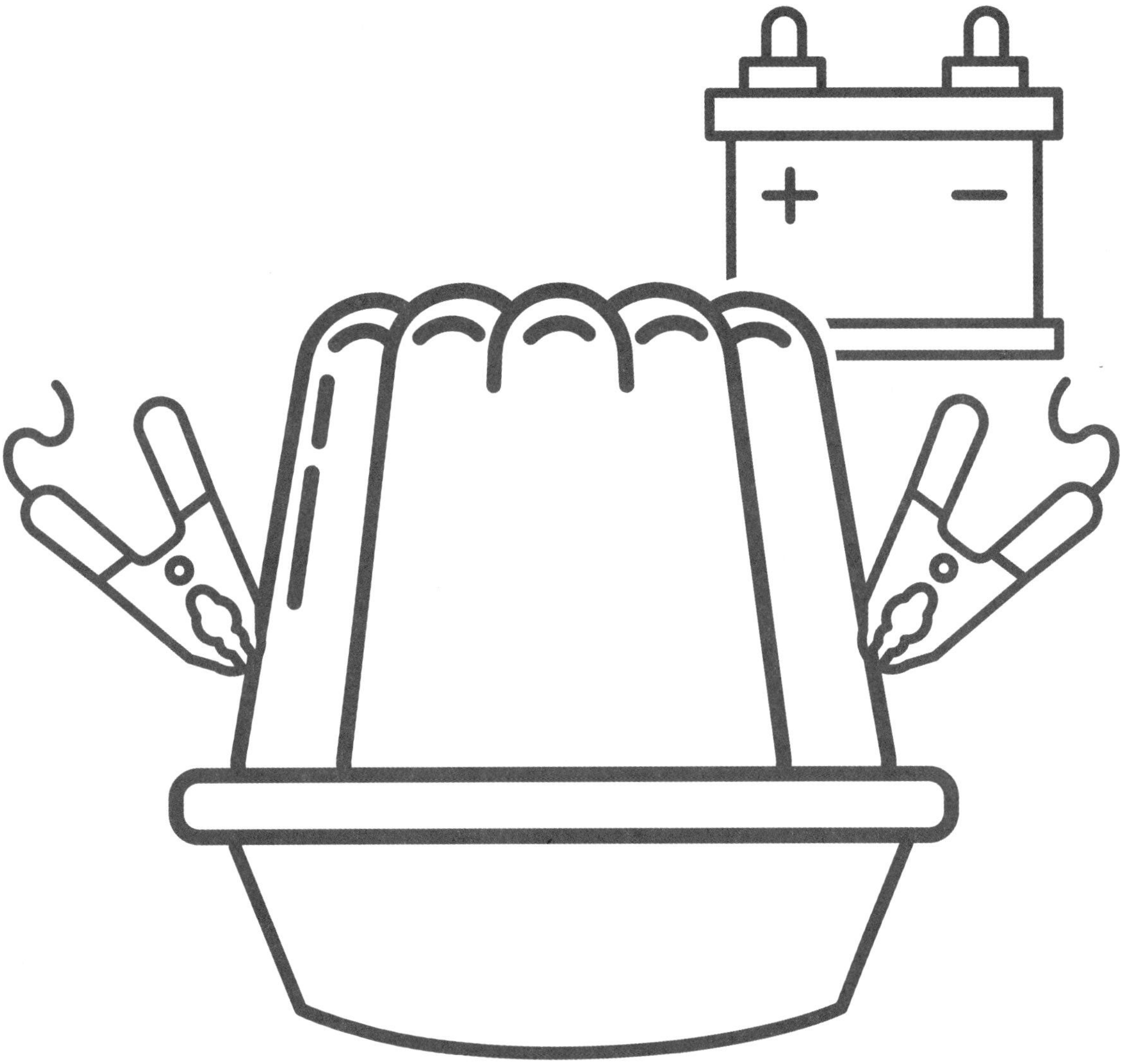

3D Glasses

Therapeutic Rationale

No modality does acceptance better than dialectical behavioral therapy (DBT), so we are going to borrow this concept with gratitude and appreciation. DBT views the world through three different perspectives: rational mind, emotional mind, and wise mind. Rational mind is all logic, no feelings—like the Vulcans from *Star Trek*. Emotional mind is the opposite, in that it's guided by feelings alone. Wise mind is really the best of both worlds, in that it incorporates both logic and emotion. In this exercise, kids will use 3D glasses as a fun and visual way to view things from a wise mind perspective.

Goals

- Learn the concepts of rational mind, emotional mind, and wise mind
- Incorporate wise mind to change clients' perspective

Materials

- Old-school red and blue lens 3D movie glasses (you can buy them in bulk online!)

Instructions

1. Give your client a brief introduction to the concept of emotional mind and rational mind, explaining that these states are like lenses through which we view the world.
2. Have your client put on a pair of 3D glasses and close the "red" eye. Ask what happens. (They will share that everything looks blue.)
3. Explain that this is like looking at the world through a purely rational mind. Ask them if that means that the entire world is actually blue. Hopefully, they will say no.
4. Now have them open the "red" eye and close the "blue" eye. Ask again what they see. (They will share that everything looks red.)
5. Explain that this is like looking at the world through a purely emotional mind. Ask them if that means that the entire world is actually red. Again, hopefully, they will say no.
6. Have them take off their 3D glasses. Tell them that this is like looking at the world through a wise mind perspective. They are not only seeing red or only seeing blue. Instead, they can see the world from a realistic perspective, as it actually is. Some things are red; some things are blue. Some things are also green, yellow, purple, or a bunch of different colors.
7. Help them search for examples in their own life where they have made use of rational mind, emotional mind, and wise mind.

Too Big to Hold

Therapeutic Rationale

Our thoughts and emotions are a normal part of being human. That being said, if we fight against them or try to force them to go away, they often get bigger . . . and bigger . . . and harder to hold. This activity uses a balloon as a metaphor to help kids understand what happens when we put too much energy into avoiding or overreacting to difficult feelings. Instead of trying to get rid of emotions, ACT teaches us to notice them, sit with them, accept them, and ultimately make space for them in a way that is manageable for us to hold onto.

Goals

- Introduce the concept of acceptance in a developmentally appropriate way
- Build insight into how avoiding emotions can make them feel bigger and harder to manage
- Begin to practice noticing emotions without trying to push them away

Materials

- One balloon per participant (e.g., clinician, client, caregiver)
- Safe space to release the balloon (secure fragile objects if inside)
- Permanent marker

Instructions

1. Introduce the balloon as a metaphor by showing the client a deflated balloon and asking, "If this balloon was a feeling, like sadness or worry, but it was small just like this balloon, could I carry it around and hold onto it?"
2. Ask the client to write a thought or emotion on the deflated balloon—ideally one they have a hard time holding onto.
3. Reinforce the idea that emotions, like this balloon, can be present without taking over. We can carry them with us without them getting in the way: "This balloon is like that feeling—it's here, it's real, but right now it's small and manageable. I can even carry it in my pocket and still go about my day."
4. Now start to gradually inflate the balloon. Notice how the thought or feeling that was written on it starts to warp and change and grow.
5. After each breath, pause and ask, "Is it getting easier or harder to hold? How clearly can you see the original thought or feeling? How easy is it to focus on everything around you while it grows?"
6. Optionally, let the balloon go and zip around the room, illustrating how emotions can "get away from us" and cause unintentional chaos, like saying or doing things we don't mean. Afterward, we often have to go pick up the pieces.

7. Explain how instead of trying to push away a thought or feeling, we can just notice it, like gently holding a small balloon. Sometimes, emotions and thoughts may grow, and that's okay, but by noticing them early, we can stay in control instead of letting them take over.
8. Wrap up by asking, "What are some ways we can make space for our thoughts and emotions without making them grow bigger and bigger?"

Guilt vs. Shame Detectives

Therapeutic Rationale

Our entire ethos as clinicians could be summed up as "Be curious, not judgmental." However, judgment often doesn't appear as obvious criticism. It can look like anger. It can look like fear. Many times, it looks like guilt or shame. Since clients often confuse guilt and shame, it is important to help them distinguish between the two: Guilt is feeling bad about something you have *done*, while shame is feeling bad about who you *are*. This activity helps clients notice and separate these emotions so they can respond with insight rather than getting stuck in self-blame.

Goals

- Get curious about emotions
- Notice thoughts without acting as though they are true

Materials

- Blank paper
- Writing utensil

Instructions

1. Introduce the concepts of guilt and shame, helping your client understand the difference. A way to remember the difference is that in a court of law, you're declared guilty, not ashamed.
2. Ask the client to write a list of things they feel guilty or ashamed about, helping them sort which are related to actions (guilt) and which are related to identity or self-worth (shame).
3. Discuss how guilt is usually tied to specific "crimes" and can motivate people to make things right, while shame often leads people to feel worthless or stuck, making it harder to heal.
4. Acknowledge that guilt can sometimes be appropriate (like after stealing a car or cheating on a test), but more often than not, it is exaggerated and inappropriate.
5. Review the client's list together. For each "crime," use a 0–10 scale to rate how much guilt or shame they feel. For example, if they stole a candy bar and rate guilt as an 8, help them see that while some guilt is appropriate (after all, they did steal!), an 8 might be too high—maybe a 3 or 4 fits better. Then discuss ways they could reduce guilt by making amends, like apologizing or replacing the candy bar.
6. Emphasize that guilt and shame should only apply to actions, not thoughts or feelings, since only actions impact others. Thoughts and feelings, no matter how uncomfortable, don't impact others unless acted upon, so they don't warrant guilt or shame. This is often a radical idea for clients that will probably take some getting used to.

Put It in Your Pocket

Therapeutic Rationale

As clinicians, we often find that the fear and distress clients feel while trying to avoid a thought or emotion is far greater than the discomfort of simply experiencing it. After all, thoughts and feelings are nothing more than chemical and electrical signals in our brains—until we give them power over us. When we stop fighting and start acknowledging what we are feeling and thinking, we can take our power back. We don't have to fix or change our thoughts and feelings in this moment—we just have to write them down and keep them in a safe place until we have the time and space to work through them later.

Goals

- Observe thoughts and feelings without trying to change them
- Reinforce the idea that acceptance means acknowledging what *is*, not approving of it

Materials

- Pocket-sized spiral notebook
- Writing utensil
- Feelings wheel (optional)

Instructions

1. Introduce the idea that thoughts and feelings only have power if we give it to them. Ask the client to give an example of a recent thought or feeling that bothered them, and talk about how it felt when they tried to fight it versus when they just noticed it.
2. Review the concept of acceptance, reinforcing the idea that acceptance doesn't mean we think that something is okay. It means acknowledging that it is the reality of the situation for the time being. Ask your client how they feel about accepting their thoughts and feelings, especially the scary ones!
3. Introduce the idea of the "Okay Book," which is a small notebook for writing down thoughts or feelings without needing to fix them right away. Emphasize that it's *not* about saying the situation is okay. It's about saying, "I'm feeling (or thinking) this . . . and that is okay."
4. Teach and practice the steps of *see it, say it*, and *okay it* in their book:
   a. **See it:** Identify the situation causing distress.
   b. **Say it:** Identify the thoughts or feelings that are causing the distress (using a feelings wheel if necessary).
   c. **Okay it:** Reframe with acceptance: "I am feeling (or thinking) this . . . and that is okay."
5. Encourage them to use their notebook regularly and to bring it to sessions. It can also be helpful to point out that the notebook is tiny; anything that is that small cannot possibly be all *that* bad.

Permission Slip

Therapeutic Rationale

Big feelings can feel overwhelming and scary, especially for younger clients. Sometimes, the fear of experiencing these emotions is even worse than the feelings themselves. This exercise provides a tangible way for kids to understand that it's okay to have big emotions and that they can learn to manage them safely instead of running away from them or letting them explode out of control. Feelings can be scary, but running from them can be scarier.

Goals

- Reduce stigma around big feelings
- Empower clients to manage big emotions in more effective ways

Materials

- *Permission Slip* worksheet
- Writing utensil

Instructions

1. Ask your client to remember a time when they had big feelings. What happened? Did they scream, cry, break things, or hit people? Did they try to hold all of their feelings inside?
2. Ask them whether they think it's okay to have big feelings. Remind them that feelings (even the big ones!) are just feelings, and it's okay to have them. They just need to give themselves a plan to deal with them safely and effectively.
3. Fill out the *Permission Slip* worksheet with your client. On the worksheet, they will:
    a. Identify a time when they experienced big emotions.
    b. Write what they were thinking and feeling at the time.
    c. Brainstorm coping skills they can use next time to feel better or stay safe.
4. Send home several blank copies of the worksheet for your client and their caregiver to complete *after* the next time they have a big feeling. Make sure the caregiver doesn't try to prompt the client to complete the worksheet *during* the big feeling. (That likely won't end well!) Instead, they should help the client regulate first and then fill it out once they are both calm.
5. Have the client bring in their completed worksheets to the next session to see what's working to help them feel better.

Permission Slip Worksheet

Complete this worksheet after you've experienced a big emotion. Fill it out once you're feeling calm, not in the middle of the moment. This helps you understand what happened, how you felt, and what you can do next time to take care of yourself in a safe way. You can do it with a caregiver or on your own!

What happened that caused you to have a big emotion?

____

____

What were you feeling at the time?

____

____

What were you thinking at the time?

____

____

What can you do about it next time?

____

____

I hereby give myself permission to feel these feelings and think these thoughts. I know that I will be okay, and that it is okay to let these feelings out in a safe way.

____________________ ____________________

Client Signature Therapist Signature

Dear Emotion . . .

Therapeutic Rationale

Emotions are messengers. Even emotions that feel tough or unhelpful, like fear, sadness, anger, or anxiety, are trying to tell us something. When we ignore them, fight with them, or try to push them away, we miss the opportunity to understand what they're trying to say. This activity helps children build a relationship with their emotions by having them write a letter *from* the emotion to themselves, and then a letter *back* to the emotion.

Goals

- Foster a sense of curiosity and compassion toward difficult emotions
- Understand the underlying purpose or function of emotions
- Externalize and respond to emotions with acceptance and care

Materials

- Blank paper
- Writing utensil

Instructions

1. Choose an emotion to work with by asking the client to think of a recent feeling that was big or uncomfortable (e.g., anxiety, anger, sadness). Help them name it clearly and explain, "Today we're going to write letters to and from this feeling, like it's a character that wants to talk to you."
2. Create a letter *from* the emotion. Ask the client to imagine they *are* the emotion, writing a letter to themselves. What would this emotion say? What is it trying to do? Guide them with questions like "Why do you [*the emotion*] show up?" "What are you afraid of?" and "How are you trying to help me, even if it doesn't always feel helpful?" Younger children can dictate this letter while you write it word for word.
3. Then create a letter *to* the emotion. What does the child want to say to this feeling? Help them respond with curiosity and kindness (e.g., "I understand why you come around," "Sometimes I wish you didn't show up so much, but I get that you're trying to protect me," "Here's what I need from you . . ."). Again, younger kids can dictate their response.
4. Ask your client what they learned about their emotions, what surprised them, how they feel about the emotion now, and how they might respond to it in the future. Reinforce that all emotions, even the uncomfortable ones, have a purpose, so it's helpful to listen to them instead of fighting them. There are no good or bad emotions!

Snake Wrangler

Therapeutic Rationale

This exercise gives voice to your client's inner experiences by creating a segmented snake that represents their thoughts and feelings. Some segments may feel big, heavy, or even sharp like fangs, while others might feel harmless or light. Just like the snake's segments, all of our thoughts and emotions are just other parts of us. No part is good or bad—they just *are*. This activity teaches kids that instead of fighting their thoughts or feelings, they can "wrangle" them with curiosity and kindness.

Goals

- Promote acceptance of all thoughts and feelings
- Build emotional literacy by naming and describing emotions
- Increase psychological flexibility by encouraging curiosity over control

Materials

- Colorful construction paper, cardstock, or cardboard
- Scissors
- Fasteners, tape, glue stick, or stapler
- Crayons, markers, colored pencils, or paint
- Craft items (e.g., googly eyes, feathers, stickers, glitter, pipe cleaners, pom poms) (optional)

Instructions

1. Cut out strips of paper to make the body of the snake. Make each one a different size, shape, and even texture. Some can be twisty, spiky, or small, just like our thoughts and feelings. You can help the client cut if needed, or precut a variety of strips before the session.
2. On each strip, have the client write or draw a thought, feeling, or even an experience. Encourage them to pick a strip size that reflects the magnitude of that thought, feeling, or experience. For example, a strong or important feeling might go on a larger strip. Encourage the client to decide which thought or feeling fits best on each strip. Ask questions to explore their choices: "I noticed you put this thought on a particularly big piece. Can you tell me more about that?" Encourage the client to decorate each piece to reflect what is written.
3. Invite the child to create the snake's head and tail however they like—maybe their snake wears a top hat, or its tail is a maraca! On the head, write something like "These are all my thoughts and feelings. Some feel tricky, but they all belong."
4. Put the snake together using tape, glue, or a stapler. If you have fasteners, use them to help the snake move and wriggle around. This is not necessary but a fun part of the flexibility.

5. After the activity, offer some reflection prompts. For example:
    - "What was one part of your snake that felt really tricky or sharp?"
    - "Have you ever tried to get rid of a tricky feeling or thought? What happened?"
    - "What do you think it means to be a good snake wrangler—someone who can wrangle all their thoughts and feelings, even the tough ones?"
    - "What helps you stay calm when your 'snake thoughts' are fighting back?"

Feelings Thermometer

Therapeutic Rationale

Sometimes, our feelings start out small, like a warm breeze or a hug, and sometimes they heat up until we feel like we're about to boil over! This activity uses a feelings thermometer to help kids recognize and track the intensity of their feelings. When they can notice and accept how "hot" their emotions are getting, they are better able to move through and with them as opposed to boiling over.

Goals

- Support mindful awareness of emotions
- Promote emotional acceptance instead of avoidance
- Create space between feelings and reactions

Materials

- *My Feelings Thermometer* worksheet
- Writing utensil
- Crayons, markers, or colored pencils

Instructions

1. Work with the child to label each level on the thermometer using the following scale:

1	2	3	4	5
Cool and Calm	Warm and Aware	Getting Toasty	Hot, Hot, Hot!	Boiling Over!

2. Ask the client to draw or write what thoughts, feelings, or situations they associate with each level on the thermometer. For example, reading peacefully might be a 1, while slamming a door might be a 5. You can use the Zones of Regulation colors as a guide (e.g., green for calm, yellow for nervous, red for out of control, and blue for low energy), but the most important thing is that the colors make sense to the child.
3. Talk about how using the thermometer is like checking the weather before getting dressed. It helps the child feel more prepared and make better choices.
4. Invite the child to use the thermometer daily, either after school or in the evening, to reflect on what happened during the day, how their emotions changed, and how they responded.
5. After the activity, offer some reflection prompts. For example:
    - "Did your temperature stay the same or change throughout the day?"
    - "What helped you the most today (e.g., person, coping skill)?"
    - "What temperature do you think you'll start tomorrow at, and why?"

My Feelings Thermometer Worksheet

Use this worksheet to check in with your feelings throughout the day. Think of your emotions like the temperature on a thermometer: Sometimes you're cool and calm, and sometimes you're starting to boil! Fill it out after school or in the evening.

Time of Day	What Was Happening?	What Was Your Temperature?	How Did You Respond?

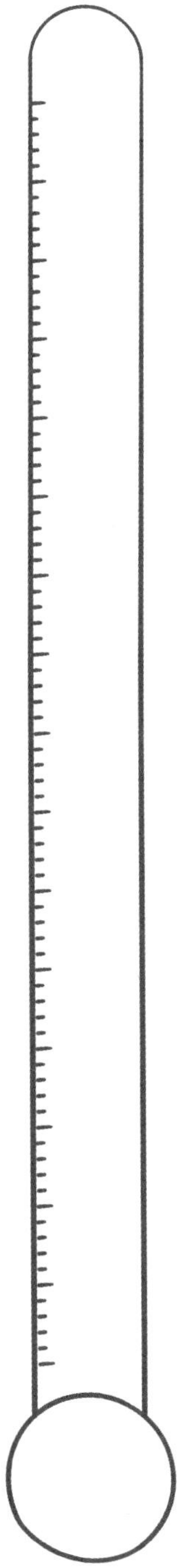

Cracks in the Sidewalk: Part 1

Therapeutic Rationale

Life is full of cracks in the sidewalk—unexpected bumps, tricky sticky thoughts, unseen pitfalls, uncomfortable feelings, and difficult memories. Sometimes, we can get so focused on avoiding these that we lose sight of the path ahead, and often, we still trip on the cracks anyway! But what if we could notice these cracks *without* letting them stop us? This activity helps kids notice the emotional and cognitive "cracks" that show up along their path. Instead of trying to step over, erase, or fix every crack, they explore what it's like to keep walking with curiosity, creativity, and compassion. This is a two-part activity, with part 2 found on page 223 in Section 5: Values.

Goals

- Accept difficult thoughts, feelings, and experiences
- Build psychological flexibility by moving toward values, even when it feels hard
- Foster curiosity and compassion for emotions and thoughts

Materials

- *Cracks in the Sidewalk* template
- Writing utensil
- Colored pencils, crayons, markers

Instructions

1. Ask the client to imagine that they are walking down a path toward something they care about (their values), but along the way, cracks in the sidewalk start to appear.
2. Help them name the "cracks" or obstacles that get in their way. These might be thoughts, feelings, memories, or experiences. Have them write these down on the *Cracks in the Sidewalk* template.
3. Ask the client, "What do you usually do when these cracks get in your way? Do you freeze, turn around, or pretend they aren't there? Do these strategies help or make it harder?"
4. Then help them brainstorm ways they could keep walking, even with the cracks there.
5. Invite the client to decorate the sidewalk and cracks with drawings, colors, or stickers as a reminder to keep going in spite of challenges.
6. As they decorate their sidewalk, remind them of the values and goals they are walking toward.

Cracks in the Sidewalk Template

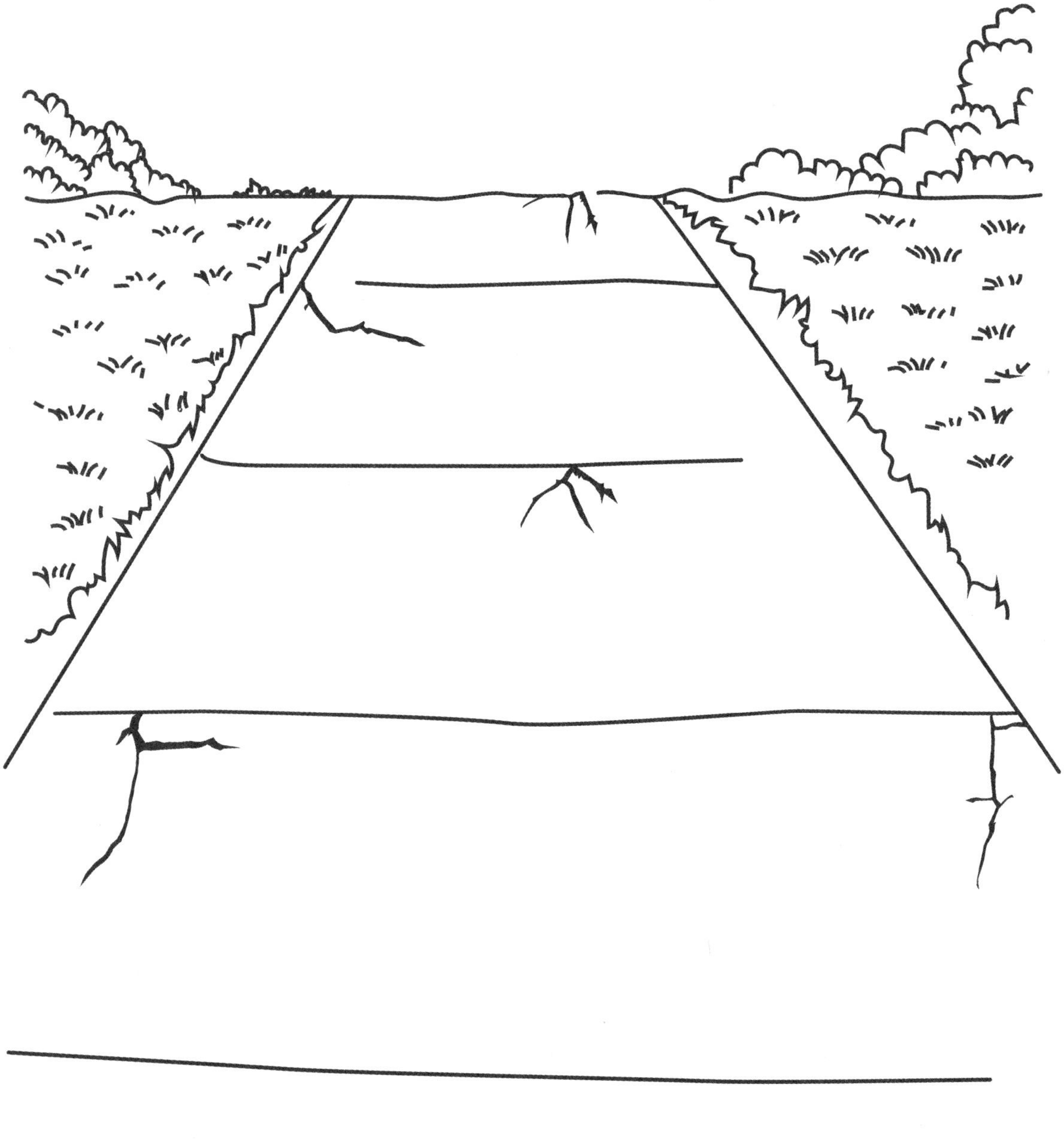

Scheduled Freakout Time

Therapeutic Rationale

We all need to freak out sometimes! When things get overwhelming, trying to hold it all back can feel like trying to plug a dam with our finger—it's only a matter of time before pressure builds and the dam bursts. Instead of trying to hold back the water, this activity teaches kids how to *channel* it down a safe and helpful path. Scheduled freakout time gives kids permission to admit that they're not okay, countering the common belief that they are not allowed to struggle or have a difficult time. This activity normalizes those feelings and reminds them that tough moments don't last forever.

Goals

- Enhance emotion regulation skills
- Reduce shame around big emotions
- Provide a safe outlet for strong emotions

Materials

- Stopwatch or timer
- Music, pillow, cozy blanket, space for movement (optional)

Instructions

1. Share the metaphor of a dam under pressure. Emotions build like water behind the wall. If we try to block them entirely, they can explode. But if we give them a channel, they can flow out safely.
2. Brainstorm with your client different ways to have a safe freakout. Some suggestions:
    - Cry while lying in bed wrapped in a cozy blanket
    - Scream in a car (alone) or into a pillow
    - Curse (with permission from a caregiver!)
    - Snuggle with a pet
    - Dance, run, or exercise intensely
    - Spend some alone time in a closet, shed, or other quiet space
3. Whatever your client decides to try, there are a couple of important things to remember:
    - They have to set a limit for their freakout. Ten or fifteen minutes is enough, but that's it. It cannot go on forever.
    - At the end of their freakout, they need to have a plan to move forward. They don't need to have a solution to what they were freaking out about, but at the very least, they have to be willing to go on with the rest of their day, even if it is not super fun to do so.
4. Remind your client to schedule this freakout anytime they need a release. Having a set time to let it out can make hard moments feel more manageable.

Emotions Tea Party

Therapeutic Rationale

This activity helps children externalize and personify their emotions, inviting them into a playful, imaginative space where feelings are seen as guests, not enemies. The goal is not to get rid of feelings but to get curious about them, noticing and accepting what they say, how they behave, and how much space they take up. This builds emotional literacy, compassion, and acceptance through a child-friendly metaphor.

Goals

- Create space between the self and emotions (self-as-context)
- Foster acceptance and openness toward all internal experiences
- Build insight into how emotions influence behavior, attention, and relationships

Materials

- Stuffed animals, dolls, or action figures
- Tea set or small table setup
- Snacks or pretend food
- Crayons, markers, or colored pencils
- Blank paper and scissors (for making nameplates)
- Hats, scarves, silly glasses, or costume items (optional)

Instructions

1. Set the scene! Invite the client to host a tea party where their emotions are the guests. Let the client pick which emotions they want to invite (e.g., worry, sadness, anger, excitement, embarrassment, joy).
2. Use dolls or stuffed animals to represent different emotions (e.g., teddy bear represents worry, unicorn represents excitement).
3. Help the child create nameplates for each emotion, letting them assign names or silly traits to each emotion (e.g., "Queen Worry has a sparkly dress but talks really fast").
4. Encourage the child to give each guest a voice and guide them with additional questions. For example:
   - "What does this emotion say at the party?"
   - "How loud are they?"
   - "Do they interrupt?"
   - "Are they bossy or shy?"
   - "How do you treat them?"

5. Observe the party! Prompt the child to notice who talks the most, who doesn't get a turn, who is kind or demanding, and who is always at the table or barely shows up.
6. After the party, offer some reflection prompts. For example:
    - "Do you *have* to do what one of your guests says?"
    - "What if you listened without obeying?"
    - "What would happen if you made room at the table for all of them?"

Feelings Forecast

Therapeutic Rationale

This take-home activity is designed to help kids recognize that emotions, like the weather, naturally shift and change—and they can acknowledge these emotions without feeling the need to control them. By tracking their "feelings forecast," kids learn to notice their emotions without judgment or avoidance. They learn that they can carry on even on stormy days. The activity also supports the development of self-as-context—the idea that "I'm noticing that I feel stormy today" is different from "I am the storm."

Goals

- Encourage emotional awareness by identifying and labeling internal states
- Foster acceptance of difficult emotions
- Increase mindfulness and flexibility over time through daily tracking

Materials

- *Feelings Forecast Chart*
- Writing utensil
- Crayons, markers, or colored pencils
- Stickers (optional)

Instructions

1. Introduce the metaphor by explaining that emotions are like the weather: They come and go, and we don't control them. Some days are sunny and others are stormy, but just like with weather, we can make choices about how we respond.
2. Help the client assign weather symbols to their most common emotions:
   a. Happy (e.g., rainbow)
   b. Sad (e.g., raindrops)
   c. Angry (e.g., tornado)
   d. Nervous (e.g., windy)
   e. Overwhelmed (e.g., thunderstorm)
   f. Calm/grateful (e.g., sunshine)
3. Explain to the client that each day, they'll draw a weather symbol (or place a sticker) on their *Feelings Forecast Chart* that matches how they felt most of the day (based on their personal weather key).
4. At the next session, review the week's weather together. Which feelings showed up the most? Did any surprise them? Which feelings lasted longer or passed quickly? Can they think of a storm that passed?

Feelings Forecast Chart

Emotions are like the weather: They come and go. Some are stormy and others are sunny. Draw a picture or symbol to show how each emotion feels for you.

Happy	Nervous	Calm
Sad	Overwhelmed	Grateful
Angry	Other: ____________	

Now use this chart to record your "weather" for each day of the week. Draw your most common emotion of the day using the following key and then answer the questions.

Week of: ______________________________

Monday	
	What did you notice about how you felt today? What did you do about it? Did your weather change during the day?

Tuesday	
	What did you notice about how you felt today? What did you do about it? Did your weather change during the day?

Wednesday	
	What did you notice about how you felt today? What did you do about it? Did your weather change during the day?

Thursday	
	What did you notice about how you felt today? What did you do about it? Did your weather change during the day?

Friday	
	What did you notice about how you felt today? What did you do about it? Did your weather change during the day?

Saturday	
	What did you notice about how you felt today? What did you do about it? Did your weather change during the day?

Sunday	
	What did you notice about how you felt today? What did you do about it? Did your weather change during the day?

Monsters on a Ship

Therapeutic Rationale

This metaphor, inspired by Dr. Russ Harris,* helps kids understand that while anxiety can feel loud and scary, it cannot actually harm them. Anxiety is like a noisy monster on their ship, not an enemy that can stop their journey. Often, people believe that the goal is to get rid of all anxiety, but that's not always possible. By accepting anxiety and moving forward despite it, kids can build resilience and learn to face their fears with courage.

Goals

- Reconceptualize how we understand anxiety
- Externalize anxiety to reduce its power
- Build resilience in the face of unpleasant emotions

Materials

- Blank paper (optional)
- Crayons, markers, or colored pencils (optional)

Instructions

1. It's story time! Ask your client to imagine they're steering a pirate ship toward an island full of treasure. But as they get closer, they hear a deep, loud, growling voice from the cargo hold, warning them not to continue. The voice threatens that if they keep going, they'll be hurt! So, they steer their ship away. The voice doesn't go away, but it quiets down . . . for a moment.
2. Your client really wants the treasure though, so they decide to slowly move back toward the island, hoping that the monster won't notice. Uh oh—it does! Now it's mad! It bursts out the cargo hold, snarling and yelling, threatening them with everything if your client doesn't turn away.
3. But your client remembers that they're a pirate! They have a sword, a cannon, and plenty of tools to protect them. So they keep sailing forward. The monster gets louder and closer, but your client realizes that it never actually touches them. It's all bark and no bite. No matter how mad it gets, *it still can't hurt them*.
4. That monster is anxiety in a nutshell. It tells us that we're not okay and that we need to be afraid, but it actually can't hurt us. It's not possible to die from a panic attack, even though it feels unpleasant and scary. It will pass.
5. **Optional:** Have the client draw their ship and their monster. They can even give the monster a silly name. One client named theirs Daisy. Now whenever they feel anxious, they just say, "Oh, Daisy is just being annoying. I'll tell her to be quiet."

---

* Dr. Russ Harris. (September 22, 2021). *Monsters on a boat* [Video]. YouTube. https://www.youtube.com/watch?v=vyxc889gQtY

Finger Trap

Therapeutic Rationale

When we feel emotions that we are not comfortable with, our first instinct is often to fight them, to try to make them stop or go away. But just like a finger trap, the more we pull and struggle, the more stuck in them we feel! This activity helps children understand that when we stop struggling—and instead turn toward our feelings with curiosity and acceptance—we often find a path forward. The finger trap becomes a powerful metaphor for emotional flexibility and a tool kids can carry with them beyond the session.

Goals

- Demonstrate how struggling with emotions can increase distress
- Pause and approach emotions with curiosity instead of judgment

Materials

- Finger trap
- Blank paper and writing utensil (optional)

Instructions

1. Introduce the finger trap and invite the client to place one finger from each hand inside. Then tell them, "Try to get your fingers out as fast as you can!"
2. Let them struggle for a while before asking, "What happened when you pulled really hard? Did it help or make things worse? How did it feel to be stuck?"
3. Guide them through the solution: "Now try something different. Instead of pulling, gently push your fingers toward each other."
4. Once they're free from the trap, ask, "What happened this time? Why do you think that worked better?"
5. Connect the metaphor to emotions by explaining that feelings can be a lot like this finger trap. When a big feeling shows up, like anger, sadness, or worry, they might want to pull away from it, but that only makes things worse. Ask, "What's a recent feeling you had that felt really big or hard to handle, like being in the finger trap? What happened when you tried to make it go away?"
6. Then offer a reframe: "What might happen if you instead slowed down and just noticed the feeling, like we did with the trap?"
7. Give the child the finger trap to take home with them as a reminder of what they learned. Encourage them to keep it somewhere accessible, like a backpack, drawer, or therapy folder. Any time a feeling shows up that they want to fight or push away, they can hold the finger trap and remember that sometimes the best way to get unstuck is to stop pulling and take a breath.

Dancing in the Rain

Therapeutic Rationale

In any difficult situation, we usually have three options: complain about it, work to change it, or work to accept it. Complaining is a great first step! It tells us what is wrong or what we're upset about. But complaining becomes a problem when we don't move on to one of the other two steps. This activity helps kids reflect on when to accept a situation, when to take action, and how to shift out of complaint mode when they're ready.

Goals

- Find joy and meaning even during difficult situations
- Strengthen psychological flexibility and the ability to see the "gray" in life
- Differentiate between acceptance and change as healthy next steps

Materials

- Blank paper
- Writing utensil

Instructions

1. With your client, split a piece of paper into three equal columns labeled "Complaint," "Work to Accept," and "Work to Change."
2. Introduce the metaphor of dancing in the rain, explaining that it's about finding ways to enjoy life even when things aren't going as planned.
3. Invite them to think of a time when they "danced in the rain," either literally or metaphorically. Together, identify their initial complaint in that situation, and whether they worked to accept or change it (or both). Then write a short note in each column to show how that situation fits into the three steps.
4. Help your client explore current complaints or frustrations in their own life. Write each one in the complaint column. Then brainstorm ways they can work to accept or change the situation. Ask them, "What would have to happen in this situation for you to be ready to move from complaining about it to one of the other two steps?"
5. Repeat the activity with as many examples as feel useful.

Beach Ball

Therapeutic Rationale

This activity uses a beach ball metaphor to help kids understand and accept their emotions. Just like a beach ball pushed underwater eventually pops back up even harder, pushing down our feelings often leads to bigger emotional reactions later. Through creative expression and guided reflection, this activity helps kids name, accept, and hold their emotions with curiosity rather than control. It's a fun, engaging way to help them move from avoidance to acceptance.

Goals

- Normalize the experience of intense or uncomfortable emotions
- Demonstrate how suppressing feelings can increase their intensity
- Notice, name, and accept emotions instead of pushing them away

Materials

- Small beach ball and tub of water
- Sticky notes
- Dry-erase marker

Instructions

1. Introduce the metaphor: "Imagine you're in a pool holding a big beach ball underwater. You're pushing and pushing, but it's hard work, and eventually the ball pops back up, sometimes even hitting you in the face! That's what it's like when we try to push down feelings like anger, sadness, or worry."
2. Ask the client if they've ever had a feeling pop up out of nowhere because they didn't talk about it.
3. Have them write or draw emotions on the beach ball (or stick notes to it). Then ask them to see what happens when they try to push the ball under water.
4. Help the client notice that the harder they push the ball down, the stronger it pushes back, sometimes even splashing more or shooting up higher.
5. Explain that, as with the beach ball, instead of pushing their feelings down, they can just hold them gently and allow them to float.
6. After the activity, offer some reflection prompts. For example:
    - "What feelings do you usually try to push down?"
    - "What happens when you do?"
    - "What would it look like to let those feelings float with you instead?"
    - "What helps you feel safe enough to talk about your feelings?"

Snowflakes

Therapeutic Rationale

Like snowflakes, our internal experiences are unique, ever-changing, and full of intricate detail. Through the act of creating and personalizing their own paper snowflakes, this activity encourages kids to observe and accept their thoughts, feelings, and ideas without judgment. The metaphor emphasizes that no two people (or internal landscapes) are exactly the same—and that complexity is something to be appreciated, not fixed or avoided. All thoughts and emotions are allowed to exist, just like snowflakes in a snowfall.

Goals

- Foster acceptance and curiosity toward internal experiences
- Support kids in identifying and labeling their emotions
- Reinforce the uniqueness and complexity of each client's inner world

Materials

- White printer or origami paper
- Scissors
- Crayons, markers, or colored pencils
- Tape or string (optional)

Instructions

1. Introduce the metaphor: "Have you ever looked at snowflakes up close? No two are the same. Each one has its own pattern, shape, and style, even though they all come from the same sky. People are like that too. We each have our own mix of thoughts, feelings, and ideas. And even *inside* of you, no two feelings are exactly alike."
2. Explain that today they'll be making snowflakes to represent the different parts of them.
3. Guide the child in folding and cutting their own unique paper snowflake. They can use pre-drawn templates or create their own designs.
4. Once the snowflake is unfolded, invite them to begin decorating it with colors, drawings, or words that represent their thoughts, feelings, and ideas—whether silly, hard, quiet, or loud. They can make one snowflake or a whole flurry, depending on time and interest.
5. After creating the snowflakes, talk together about what they included:
    a. "Which feelings showed up in your snowflake?"
    b. "Do some thoughts or feelings take up more space than others?"
    c. "If these flakes were falling in your mind, what would the weather feel like?"
6. Highlight the idea that each snowflake is allowed to be just as it is, no fixing, no hiding.
7. **Optional:** After creating the snowflakes, use tape or string to display them in your room.

Strengths Spotting

Therapeutic Rationale

This activity helps kids recognize and accept all parts of themselves, with a particular focus on the positive. As clinicians, we know that people don't often come knocking on our doors because things are going well, which means it can be easy for clients to lose sight of all of the amazing things that make them unique and wonderful. Taking a mindful moment to notice all those strengths can foster self-awareness, compassion, and a more flexible self-view. This activity is especially helpful for kids who struggle with low self-esteem, black-and-white thinking, or emotional avoidance.

Goals

- Increase awareness and acceptance of personal strengths
- Challenge self-critical thoughts
- Promote a flexible and values-based self-concept

Materials

- Blank paper
- Writing utensil
- Stopwatch or timer
- Word bank (optional)

Instructions

1. Introduce the activity by explaining that we sometimes forget all of the many different, wonderful parts of ourselves that make us who we are. It can be easy to focus on the things we want to improve, but if we don't also take the time to notice the positive, quirky, silly, or even neutral parts of ourselves, we can get lost in the challenges. This activity is about *noticing* all of those pieces, especially the ones we may not usually think of as strengths.
2. Set a timer for one minute and ask the client to write down as many words that come to mind that make them uniquely themselves. These can be any traits, qualities, or roles that best represent them, like loud, funny, silly, goofy, athletic, baseball player, honest, swimmer, and so on. Encourage them not to overthink their responses. If needed, provide a word bank to help them get started.
3. Once the minute is up, review the list together. Ask the client to reflect on which traits surprised them, which ones feel most true today, and whether any feel hard to accept.

Describe Yourself

Therapeutic Rationale

This activity guides clients in taking a mindful pause to notice, explore, and accept all parts of themselves—not just what they show the world, but also the parts they're still figuring out. By imagining themselves as the main character in a movie or story, they can externalize and observe their identity with curiosity, playfulness, and compassion. This reduces self-judgment and increases acceptance of their thoughts, feelings, and traits as meaningful parts of their ongoing journey.

Goals

- Promote mindful self-awareness and self-compassion
- Encourage flexible thinking about traits, emotions, and internal experiences
- Support a clear, values-based sense of identity

Materials

- Blank paper
- Writing utensil
- Crayons, markers, or colored pencils (optional)
- Craft items (e.g., stickers, glitter, glue) (optional)

Instructions

1. Explain to the client that they're going to create a character bio—as if they are the star of their own movie or book. Emphasize that this is their story, and they get to decide what to share and what to skip.
2. Use the following prompts to help them write their bio:
   a. "What words describe your personality? Feel free to look back at your *Strength Spotting* activity for ideas!"
   b. "What thoughts, feelings, or experiences do you carry around with you every day? How do they shape your character's journey?"
   c. "What are some quirks or cool facts about your character?"
   d. "What matters most to your character? What do they love to do or stand up for?"
   e. "What are they working on or trying to get better at?"
   f. "What goals, hopes, and dreams does your character have for their story?"
3. When they finish their bio, invite them to take a few deep breaths and reflect on what they have written. Explain that this is just the start of their story because each new chapter is still being written. While it's important to notice and accept what is already on the page, they can also take meaningful actions to make sure the next chapters of their story align with their values and goals.
4. **Optional:** Allow them to decorate their bio with colors, stickers, or other crafts.

Surf's Up

Therapeutic Rationale

This activity uses the metaphor of waves to help kids build awareness and acceptance of their emotions over time. By noticing how emotions rise, crest, and fall like waves, children can practice riding out intense feelings instead of avoiding them or letting the "waves" knock them down.

Goals

- Build mindful awareness and acceptance of emotions as they rise and fall like waves
- Use visualization to stay grounded during big emotional "waves"
- Enhance emotion regulation skills

Materials

- Computer with speakers (optional)

Instructions

1. Explain that emotions are like waves. When things feel particularly challenging, our emotions can feel bigger and scarier, as if they're trying to knock us down. But instead of standing there and letting the waves knock us down, we can pick up our surfboard and ride them out.
2. Guide the client to visualize this metaphor:

   "Imagine you're standing on a warm, sandy beach. You can hear the waves in the distance. You pick up your surfboard—it can look however you want. Maybe it has glitter, fire stripes, or your favorite animal on it. You walk toward the water and step onto the board.

   A wave begins to rise—it's a small feeling at first. You feel it in your body. Maybe it's excitement or worry. You hop onto your board and ride the wave. As it gets taller, the feeling gets stronger. Your heart might beat a little faster, your tummy might feel wobbly. That's okay. Just notice it.

   The wave reaches its peak, the biggest part of the feeling. You feel it fully. You ride with it. You don't fall or fight it. You're just riding and breathing.

   And then . . . the wave starts to fall. The feeling begins to change. It might crash gently or louder, but it's moving. The ocean is always moving. You're still here, still steady, still riding.

   Finally, the wave pulls back into the sea. The big feeling softens and fades. You hop off your board and stand on the shore again. You did it. You rode the wave. And it passed."

3. You can also show a video or audio clip of ocean waves to the client to add to the experience.
4. Encourage the client to remember that anytime they notice their emotions or thoughts getting too big, they can picture themselves getting on their surfboard and riding it out. It's a skill they can use anytime, anywhere.

Thought Clouds: Part 1

Therapeutic Rationale

Our minds are like the sky: sometimes clear and sunny, sometimes stormy and dark, and often filled with all kinds of clouds. Likewise, our thoughts and emotions drift through our minds just like clouds: Some are light and fluffy, some are heavy and gray, and some might even feel like tornadoes. Mindfulness can help us notice these clouds without getting caught up in them. We learn that all clouds belong in the sky, and all thoughts and feelings can come and go without needing to change or fix them. We can simply observe them without having to run toward or away from them.

Goals

- Practice mindful, nonjudgmental awareness of thoughts and feelings
- Encourage acceptance of thoughts and feelings without needing to change them
- Reinforce that all internal experiences are temporary and natural

Materials

- Blank paper
- Writing utensil
- Crayons, markers, or colored pencils
- Pre-drawn cloud outlines for younger children (optional)

Instructions

1. Explain that the mind is like the sky. Thoughts and feelings float through it like clouds. Some clouds are soft and gentle, others stormy or scary, some big and loud, and others small and quiet. But they all belong in the sky.
2. Invite the child to draw a large sky across their paper and fill it with different clouds representing thoughts or feelings they've had this week. Suggest fluffy clouds for gentle or happy thoughts, dark clouds for sadness or anger, and swirling tornado clouds for overwhelming or scary thoughts. Encourage them to write a thought or feeling inside each cloud.
3. Review the drawing together, asking which clouds take up the most space, which ones are easier to sit with, which ones feel hard to have, and which surprised them, if any.
4. Introduce mindful noticing by explaining that just like we can look up at the sky and notice clouds drifting by without trying to push them away, we can do the same with our thoughts and feelings. We don't need to make the storm clouds leave. We can just watch them, knowing they'll pass.
5. Wrap up by asking what it would feel like to let their clouds come and go, instead of trying to change them. After, you can close with a mindful breath or visualization, such as imagining a gentle wind slowly moving the clouds across the sky.

Thought Clouds: Part 2

Therapeutic Rationale

This activity extends the cloud metaphor by providing kids with a real-world grounding experience. Stepping outside and mindfully observing the clouds—noticing how some dissipate, some move faster than others, and some merge with others—reinforces the idea that all thoughts and feelings, like clouds, are temporary. In addition, human beings are designed to spend time outside. Fresh air, sunlight, and connection to nature naturally help the body and mind feel more settled.

Goals

- Reinforce acceptance by observing the temporary nature of thoughts and feelings
- Practice grounding and remaining present in the moment
- Notice internal experiences as a means of grounding

Materials

- Safe space to sit or lie down with a view of the sky
- Blanket (optional)

Instructions

1. Bring your client outside and find a comfortable, quiet spot to sit or lie on the ground together. Let them know that you'll be watching some clouds. There's no need to rush or talk the whole time. There will probably be more than a few periods of silence during this activity. Unlike some of the other activities in this book, the point is to remain present more than anything else.
2. As the clouds float by, prompt your client to notice different things about the clouds (e.g., "I notice that those clouds are really wispy," "I notice that those clouds are moving slowly," "I notice that those clouds are higher up").
3. Ask your client to notice what they are experiencing internally as well (e.g., "I notice that I am feeling calmer," "I notice that I am feeling sad," "I notice that I am hungry").
4. Relate this back to *Thought Clouds: Part 1* by reminding your client that just like clouds, our thoughts and emotions drift in and out. Even storm clouds eventually pass.
5. After you've allowed ample time for cloud watching, end your time outside and discuss how your client can incorporate this practice into their own life. Whenever they need a moment of calm, they simply need to take a few minutes to observe the sky and imagine their thoughts or emotions drifting by like clouds.

Making Oobleck

Therapeutic Rationale

Have you ever tried to *not* think or feel something? It usually has the opposite effect in that whatever you are trying to avoid tends to stick around longer. For example, if I told you that no matter what, you could not smile, and you *had* to stop yourself from smiling . . . what would happen? Go ahead, try it! No smiling. Zero. Zilch. Is that a lip twitch? Don't do it! I'm warning you! Oh no, a smile! Trying to control our emotions often ends the same way. So much of our distress occurs when we try to control or suppress our thoughts and feelings. Instead, we can practice simply acknowledging what we are experiencing, noticing it, and letting it just exist—without running from it or fusing with it. Oobleck is a fun, hands-on way for kiddos to visualize this.

Goals

- Build comfort with thoughts and feelings rather than resisting them
- Support grounding during moments of panic
- Notice thoughts and feelings without getting sucked in or controlled by them

Materials

- Corn starch
- Water
- Mixing bowl
- Sandwich baggie
- Food dye (optional)

Instructions

1. Tell your client that you'll be doing an experiment together, but don't explain what is going to happen just yet.
2. Have the client mix together approximately two parts corn starch to one part water. Add food coloring if desired. You will know that it has been mixed correctly when it flows gently when left alone and becomes firm when pressure is applied to it.
3. Once it has been mixed, give the client time to touch, handle, and play with the oobleck. Ask them what they notice about the oobleck and what is strange about it.
4. Ask the client if there are any similarities between the oobleck and their thoughts or emotions. As with the oobleck, when we simply notice our thoughts and feelings, they can flow freely, but if we try to push and pull them in a particular direction, they harden and become inflexible. Talk about any instances where they have noticed this in their own life.
5. Brainstorm strategies to help the client notice when they are becoming rigid or trying to force their thoughts and feelings. Remind them of their coping and grounding skills.
6. Give the client the oobleck in a sealed baggie as a tactile reminder of today's session.

Rushing Through the Rain

Therapeutic Rationale

This activity helps kids understand that resisting or rushing through uncomfortable feelings often leads to greater distress, just like running through the rain can actually get us wetter. By encouraging clients to pause and notice moments of discomfort with openness and curiosity—rather than avoidance or urgency—they can reduce reactivity to uncomfortable internal states.

Goals

- Increase emotional tolerance through mindful awareness
- Normalize discomfort as part of the human experience
- Encourage slower, more intentional responses to stress

Materials

- Blank paper
- Writing utensil
- Crayons, markers, or colored pencils

Instructions

1. Describe how running in heavy rain usually makes us wetter because raindrops hit us from more angles: "Have you ever been caught in the rain? Imagine your parent's car is all the way across the parking lot and it is absolutely pouring outside! Your first instinct is likely to make a run for it. But, when we do that, we actually end up getting hit with more raindrops because they hit us from the top and the front. Funny enough, if we slow down and just walk at a normal pace, we oftentimes will get less wet."
2. Ask your client what helps them pause or slow down when their brain is telling them to run. For example, this might include taking deep breaths or counting to ten.
3. Invite your client to draw themselves standing in the rain. As they create their drawing, invite them to think about what the raindrops represent—perhaps they are worries, anger, sadness, or pressure. Ask whether they are running in the drawing or pausing to breathe and stay calm. Let them know it's okay to add an umbrella or raincoat if they want. We all need some extra support every now and then!

Sticky Notes

Therapeutic Rationale

This activity is designed to help kids notice when they're judging—and learn to set aside those judgments whenever possible. Judgment can show up in many different ways: through assumptions, anger, anxiety, and especially through labeling. Instead of judging thoughts, feelings, or experiences based on what we fear they might be—or what we fear they could become—we want to support kids in simply noticing them for what they are.

Goals

- Reframe judgments into neutral observations
- Emphasize the importance of curiosity and playfulness

Materials

- Sticky notes
- Writing utensil

Instructions

1. Lead a discussion about judging (and fearing) thoughts and emotions. Ask your client about specific times in their life when they've judged events, people, thoughts, experiences, or emotions. Explore examples when those judgments turned out to be partly or entirely inaccurate. Remember to make sure the discussion is developmentally appropriate; this content can be pretty abstract!
2. Tell your client that you are going to play a game. Give them the sticky notes and ask them to label objects in your office. The labels should be simple and neutral—for example, "pencil," "chair," "book," and so on.
3. Next, tell them that you want to change the labels. Have them re-label each object with its scariest possible outcome or use (within reason—nothing too violent!). For example, "book" could become "hand smasher," and "power outlet" could become "electrocutor."
4. When they're done, ask the client what each version of the activity felt like and how the experiences differed. Which labels seem more useful? Lead this back to a discussion about thoughts and feelings, and how we can approach them with curiosity (like the first set of labels) instead of judgment (like the second set).
5. Practice helping the client reframe some of their own judgments into more neutral and curious terms.

SECTION 2

Cognitive Defusion

Defusion in the context of ACT refers to unhooking from unhelpful thoughts and feelings. When we identify too closely with a thought or a feeling, we begin to assume that the thought or feeling is an accurate reflection of the world. That is seldom the case and can lead to tremendous distress.

Instead, we want to practice putting some space between ourselves and our thoughts and feelings, which may sound counterintuitive, depending on your theoretical orientation. After all, isn't it our job to get folks to examine their thoughts and feelings as closely as they can in an effort to gain insight? Our only response to that is a question: If you wanted to understand the migration patterns of birds, would you use a microscope? Sometimes, we get too involved, too invested in what we are feeling and thinking. We miss the forest for the trees. When we can put away the microscope, it allows us to sit for a moment and notice our thoughts and feelings. We can observe them without becoming obsessed with them or scared of them.

Some kids will be more naturally gifted at this than others. That's okay! It takes practice. You might have them start by noticing some of their more innocuous thoughts and feelings as practice. "Huh. I'm noticing that it's cold out." "I'm noticing that I'm hungry." "I'm noticing that I am feeling depressed after the Phillies were eliminated from the playoffs again." (The pain of Philadelphia sports fandom does not make for easy cognitive defusion!) Practice doesn't make perfect, because the goal is never perfection; it's progress.

Helium Balloons

Therapeutic Rationale

This activity introduces the concept of defusion in a visual and experiential way by using helium balloons to symbolize thoughts, feelings, or memories that clients often become "fused" with. It helps kids externalize and observe their internal experiences from a distance, seeing that while their thoughts and feelings still exist, they don't have to carry the same weight or influence. As children let go of the balloon, they can witness how something that once felt big can shrink with distance and perspective. It's not about erasing thoughts, but changing their relationship to them.

Goals

- Introduce the concept of defusion
- Externalize challenging thoughts or feelings to practice defusing from them

Materials

- Helium tank
- Balloons (preferably biodegradable if done outdoors)
- Permanent marker
- Safe space to release the balloons

Instructions

1. Briefly explain what defusion means in ACT and how it helps us "unhook" from thoughts and feelings instead of getting caught up in them. We can simply notice and watch them "float away," much like a balloon.
2. Head outside if possible, and inflate and tie off the first balloon. From here, help the client give voice to the thought, emotion, or experience they are going to practice defusing from.
3. Using a marker, have the client write the thought, emotion, or experience on the balloon while you hold it, or write it for them if needed.
4. Have the client hold onto the balloon for a moment without letting go. Ask them to feel and think about what they wrote. When they are ready, invite them to gently let the balloon go and imagine unhooking from the thought, feeling, or experience at the same time.
5. Guide the client in noticing that as the balloon gets smaller, it still exists and is still real, but it becomes a much smaller part of their view as it floats away. Explain that the same can be true of the thoughts, feelings, and experiences they unhook from.
6. Help the client process what it feels like to watch what they wrote down float away and not feel so big anymore. Remind them that they can do this activity anytime by picturing the balloon in their mind and watching it float away.
7. This activity can be repeated several times with different thoughts or feelings, and it can also be revisited as needed across multiple sessions.

Perspective Detective

Therapeutic Rationale

This activity introduces the foundational ACT principle that thoughts are not facts through the use of a fun, kid-friendly metaphor: being a detective. Many kids assume that their thoughts are always true (e.g., "I can't do this," "Nobody likes me"), but this activity helps them take a step back, gather evidence, and explore alternative perspectives. By taking on the role of a detective, they learn to examine their thoughts with curiosity instead of certainty, increasing psychological flexibility and reducing automatic, unhelpful fusion with self-critical or anxious beliefs.

Goals

- Introduce the idea that thoughts are not always true, even if they feel strong
- Practice gathering evidence for and against a belief
- Reduce unhelpful cognitive fusion by slowing down automatic thinking

Materials

- *Perspective Detective* worksheet
- Writing utensil

Instructions

1. Introduce the activity: "Sometimes, we believe our thoughts right away, like they're 100 percent true, just because they popped into our head. But thoughts aren't always facts. That's why we're going to become Perspective Detectives today! Detectives don't just jump to conclusions. They look for clues, ask questions, and check the evidence. We're going to do the same with your thoughts. When a thought shows up, we'll look at it from all angles to see if it's trying to trick you or tell you something helpful."
2. Have the child write down a stressful or worrisome thought exactly as it appears in their mind on the *Perspective Detective* worksheet. Encourage them to use this template as you proceed through the following steps together.
3. Determine whether the thought is a fact or a feeling by asking, "Can you prove this thought is true with evidence, or is this just how you feel right now?" Explain that while feelings are real, they are not always accurate reflections of reality.
4. Determine the evidence *for* the thought by asking, "What makes this thought seem true? Can you think of any examples or clues that support it?" (e.g., "I've messed up before").
5. Gather the evidence *against* the thought by asking, "What makes this thought less true or not always true? Can you find examples or clues that don't support this thought?" (e.g., "I practiced a lot," "My teacher said I did well last time").

6. Review all of the evidence and ask, "Does this thought still feel 100 percent true?" Explain that by taking on the role of a detective and slowing down their thinking, they can notice their thoughts without automatically believing or acting on them.

Perspective Detective Worksheet

Put on your detective hat! Look for clues to determine whether your thought is 100 percent true.

What is the thought?

Is it a fact or a feeling?

What's the evidence *for* the thought?

What's the evidence *against* the thought?

Three True Questions Decision Tree

Therapeutic Rationale

Ultimately, much of our psychological distress comes from feeling helpless or out of control. Although there are a variety of interventions to help kids figure out what they can and can't control, they often stop short of addressing the bigger question: What do we do after we realize we can't control something yet still feel distressed about it? This decision tree offers a simple visual way to help kids shift their perspective and respond more flexibly.

Goals

- Learn about and practice cognitive defusion when appropriate
- Practice incorporating ideas of acceptance as it relates to lack of control

Materials

- *Decision Tree* handout

Instructions

1. Explain that distress often comes from wanting to control something that we can't. Ask the client to identify a situation that is currently causing them stress, worry, or frustration. You may want to ask questions like "What about this situation would you like to control but feel like you cannot?" "What is bothering you so much about this situation?" or "What are you worried will happen as a result of this?"
2. Connect the concept of control to acceptance by explaining that acceptance does not mean liking or approving of a situation—it simply means acknowledging that it is going on. It's about meeting life on life's terms.
3. Share the *Decision Tree* handout, and walk through each of the three questions using their example:
    a. Is what you're thinking true?
        - If it is not true ⇒ No worries! No need to be upset about it.
        - If it is true ⇒ Go on to question 2.

    b. If it is true, is it as big of a deal as you are making it out to be?
        - If it is true but not as big of a deal ⇒ Fantastic! No need to be bothered by it.
        - If it is true and as big of a deal as you think ⇒ Go on to question 3.

    c. If it is true *and* as big of a deal as you're making it out to be, is there anything you can do to change it?
        - If yes ⇒ Wonderful! You do not have to be upset because you can work to change the situation.

- If no ⇒ Time to practice acceptance because being upset about it for the rest of your life probably will not help.
  - If you have arrived at this prompt, then brainstorm how to accomplish that acceptance with your client.

4. Repeat the process with additional real-life scenarios, ideally over the course of multiple sessions. Give the client a printout to take home with them, and encourage them to use it anytime they need to defuse from distressing thoughts.

Decision Tree Handout

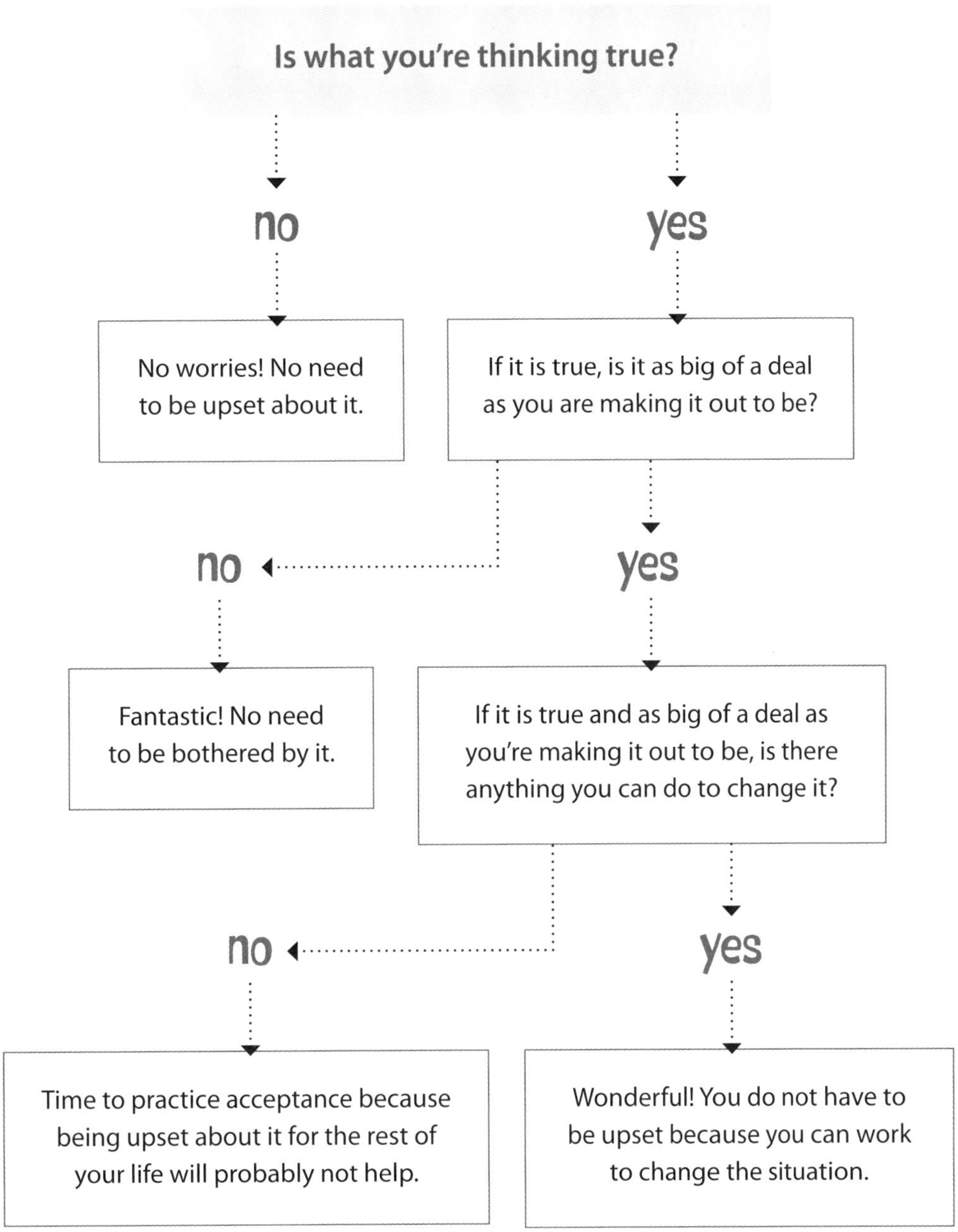

Bouncy Balls

Therapeutic Rationale

In our experience, folks often equate cognitive defusion with doing anything you can to *not* think of something. Have you ever tried to *not* think of something? It's almost impossible! If we said that no matter what, you absolutely cannot think of a giant purple elephant, what is likely to be the first thing that pops into your head? Of course, a giant purple elephant. Cognitive defusion is different. Instead of running from our thoughts, we practice setting them aside and allowing them to simply *be*, which allows us to find far more peace.

Goals

- Practice cognitive defusion in a hands-on way
- Notice thoughts without engaging with them or avoiding them

Materials

- Small bouncy balls

Instructions

1. Give your client a bouncy ball and invite them to carefully bounce it or toss it up and catch it. What do they notice? Is it easy? Is it hard?
2. Now ask them to throw the ball so it stays far away from them—for example, by throwing it against a wall (or another hard, safe surface). Predictably, the ball will bounce back at them!
3. Next, ask them to brainstorm another way they can move as far away from the ball as possible while staying in the room. The goal is to help them figure out that if they gently place the ball in one corner of your office, they can freely move to the opposite corner without being pursued by a bouncing ball.
4. Point out that the ball is still there, ready for them to pick up and engage with whenever they are ready, but they are not being hounded by it.
5. Ask them to consider how the bouncy ball is like a thought or emotion. When they try to throw it away forcefully, it often comes bouncing back in an unanticipated and undesired ways. If they instead set it down gently and walk away until they are ready to engage with it, they will have far greater success.
6. Invite them to reflect on times in their life when they have "thrown the ball" versus "gently placed the ball." Help them brainstorm strategies to practice gently setting down their thoughts and emotions in the future.

Movie Trailer

Therapeutic Rationale

Much of our mental and emotional anguish comes not from our experiences, but from our thoughts and feelings about our experiences. Our minds create "stories" about what happens, which is why some people are able to be "okay" in spite of tremendous adversity, while other people struggle with seemingly insignificant barriers in their lives. This activity helps kids take a step back, notice the stories they are telling themselves, and practice choosing a different perspective. Using the metaphor of a recut movie trailer, they can see that the same events can feel scary, funny, or exciting depend how they choose to frame them. By reediting their perspective (or "trailer"), they can defuse from upsetting thoughts and respond to challenges more flexibly.

Goals

- Take a hopeful perspective instead of a pessimistic one
- Find humor in situations as a means of emotional regulation

Materials

- Computer with speakers

Instructions

1. Pull up YouTube on your computer and ask your client if they have ever seen a movie trailer. Explain that trailers are the "story" the director tells about a movie—they can make one movie look either scary, funny, or exciting.
2. Search for a "recut movie trailer" for a movie your client has seen. Watch the trailer together and point out any funny or surprising edits (you may want to prewatch it if possible), and invite them to do the same. What do they notice about the trailer? What is different about it compared to the original film? What made it different?
3. Steer the conversation toward the idea that the movie itself didn't change—it is just our perspective (the trailer) that changed.
4. Explain that our life stories are often guided by "and therefore . . ." statements (e.g., "I'm really scared about a test at school, *and therefore* I'm definitely going to fail and there is nothing that I can do").
5. However, we can reedit those statements much like we could a movie trailer: "I'm really scared about a test at school, *and therefore* I'm definitely going to ask my parents to get me a tutor."
6. Connect this to the client's life by asking, "What part of your life feels like a horror movie right now? How might you recut the trailer to make it look more like a comedy?"

Video Game Boss Music

Therapeutic Rationale

Cognitive defusion is about changing the context in which we are viewing our thoughts and feelings rather than trying to fight them. A fun way to help kiddos understand this concept is through video games and movies. Most kids understand that when the music speeds up and becomes scarier, it means that a bad guy is about to strike! Sometimes, life can feel just like that—the "music" in our heads speeds up and becomes more intense, making challenging moments feel bigger than they are. The goal of this activity is to help kids recognize that they are allowed to change the music that is playing in their minds, making stressful situations easier to handle.

Goals

- Practice cognitive defusion in a relatable, engaging way
- Find humor and perspective to disengage from unhelpful thoughts

Materials

- Computer with speakers
- Video game system (optional)

Instructions

1. Ask your client if they have ever watched a movie or played a video game. They will almost certainly say yes (and they may also give you a funny look!). Then ask what happens in the game to indicate that a big boss fight is about to happen. They should be able to tell you (with a little prompting) that the music becomes faster or more intense.
2. Explore how that music makes them feel. They may feel nervous, scared, excited, happy, or something else entirely.
3. If they mention feeling nervous or scared, ask what they are afraid may happen next. Their response will probably have something to do with a fear of losing the game.
4. Ask whether the big boss fight would be as scary without the music. You can experience this with them in several ways:
   - Bring in a portable video game system and play it in session with the sound off.
   - Watch a scary (but appropriate) movie trailer that has been recut to be humorous.
5. Discuss how removing or changing the music changes the experience.
6. Connect this with real life by asking the client to consider when the "music" in their life speeds up, making them feel nervous, scared, or stressed. Explore what that is like for them and what kinds of situations trigger it. A little self-disclosure may be helpful here: "I know what that's like. I feel like the music speeds up for me sometimes too."
7. Then ask them what kind of music they would like to play instead, and discuss how this can make the situation feel more manageable.

Hall of Mirrors

Therapeutic Rationale

In ACT, we recognize that our emotional experiences are not inherently good or bad; instead, we consider whether they are helpful or unhelpful. For example, fear can be helpful when it serves to protect us, just like happiness can occasionally lead us into trouble! However, when we are overwhelmed by our experiences, it's easy to panic and feel like *all* of our emotions are unhelpful. This activity helps kids visualize what it feels like to be overwhelmed and then practice grounding themselves, noticing what their emotions are trying to tell them, and finding a path forward.

Goals

- Practice grounding and noticing emotions
- Engage in a guided visualization to understand and manage the feeling of being overwhelmed

Materials

- Computer with speakers (optional)

Instructions

1. Ask your client if they know what a hall of mirrors is and if they have ever been in one. If not, watch videos together on YouTube showing people navigating a hall of mirrors. Encourage your client to notice how confusing it can be to find the way out.
2. Discuss what they think it might feel like to get lost in a hall of mirrors. Connect this to times in their life by asking them to describe situations where they were panicking, overwhelmed, or stuck—like they were "bouncing off mirrors" without finding a way forward.
3. Guide your client through a grounding visualization. Invite them to think of one particular moment when they feel panicked or overwhelmed—just like being trapped in a hall of mirrors—then have them take a deep breath and pause. Ask them to notice where the mirrors are around them, where they are standing, and to focus on the ground beneath their feet. Explain that even in the midst of confusion or panic, they can start to see a path forward by slowing down and paying attention to what is real.
4. Help your client apply this grounding technique to their own life moving forward. Discuss how they can recognize when they are "bouncing off mirrors" (feeling overwhelmed or panicked) and how they can pause, recenter themselves, and get back on track when emotions become too overwhelming.

Healthiness Spectrum

Therapeutic Rationale

The antithesis of psychological flexibility is black-and-white thinking, which children and adolescents can be quite skilled at! They struggle to see the gray, particularly when it comes to moderation. This activity provides a visual tool to help kids practice finding those shades of gray and reframe decisions not as "healthy" or "unhealthy," but as existing on a spectrum. We have purposefully eliminated the term *unhealthy* from the spectrum because it is a matter of perspective. Instead, the focus is on seeing things on a scale of healthy, less healthy, or healthier.

Goals

- Find nuance and move away from all-or-nothing thinking
- Reframe extreme examples in search of a healthier alternative

Materials

- *Healthiness Spectrum* handout

Instructions

1. Begin by asking your client "How do you know if something is healthy or unhealthy?" Give them the space to respond, and encourage them to think critically about their answer.
2. Use gentle, probing questions to expand their definition beyond the binary of healthy/unhealthy. Ultimately, you want to collaborate toward the following definition: Healthiness exists on a spectrum and is influenced by three factors:
   a. "How much good or bad is this doing for my body?"
   b. "How much good or bad is this doing for my mind/soul?"
   c. "How often am I doing this?"
3. Use the *Healthiness Spectrum* handout to place different decisions on the spectrum and talk through the reasoning behind each placement. An example that we often reference involves eating candy. If we ate candy all day long, every single day, it might feel satisfying to our mind/soul, but our bodies might feel tired and not so great. This would probably be rated as "a lot less healthy" on our spectrum. On the other hand, if we never ate candy ever again, our bodies would feel okay but our mind/soul would feel like we're missing out on something fun. That, too, would fall under "a lot less healthy," as we certainly do not want to live in a world without candy! But if we eat candy sometimes, both our body and mind/soul can still feel good, so it would go under the "healthier" or "healthiest" category.
4. Continue to apply this spectrum to examples from your client's life, looking for extremes, and then find the middle ground that belongs under "healthier" or "healthiest" range. Encourage your client to hang up a copy of this spectrum somewhere visible to remind them to balance their choices in the future.

Healthiness Spectrum Handout

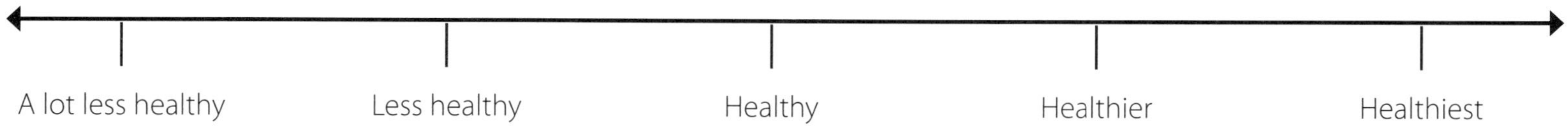

Smashing Playdough

Therapeutic Rationale

This activity provides a hands-on way for kids to practice defusion. By using playdough, kids can physically unhook from a difficult thought, feeling, or experience and then literally reshape it into something new. The act of smashing and rebuilding allows them to learn that while their thoughts and feelings are real, they are also malleable, impermanent, and not all-powerful—meaning they can defuse from them.

Goals

- Reinforce the idea that thoughts and feelings can change form and lose intensity
- Foster agency and empowerment by allowing clients to choose where to focus their energy

Materials

- Playdough or modeling clay (multiple colors if available)
- Flat workspace or tray

Instructions

1. Explain the activity to your client: "We're going to use playdough today to represent a thought, feeling, or experience that's been bothering you—something that has felt hard to unstick from. Then, we'll *smash it*—not to destroy it, but to show that it doesn't have to stay that way forever. You can reshape it and change its form. This will help you practice defusing from the thought, feeling, or experience so you can focus your time and energy on the things that matter to you."
2. Invite the client to use playdough to create a symbol, creature, or object that represents a thought, feeling, or experience they want to work with. Examples might include a worry monster, a tangled ball of stress, or a shape that feels "heavy."
3. Encourage them to flatten, squish, or smash the playdough gently but intentionally. As they mold the dough, say "Notice what happens when you change its shape. The thought still exists—it's just not the same as it was before. You're in charge of what you do with it now."
4. Next, invite the client to reshape the smashed dough into something that represents a value, goal, or something they enjoy. This could be a heart (for love), a star (for hope), a sun (for happiness), or a dance shoe (for passion). Discuss how it feels to turn something difficult into something meaningful.

5. After the activity, offer some reflection prompts. For example:
    - "What did your first creation represent?"
    - "What changed when you smashed it?"
    - "How did it feel to make something new?"
    - "How can you remember this next time a tough thought shows up?"

Skill Practice and Application

Lost in Translation

Therapeutic Rationale

This activity uses the metaphor of a translator to help kids understand that thoughts are not absolute truths or commands—they are simply words. By translating a "sticky" thought into different languages—whether real or invented—children can notice how the weight, tone, and *stickiness* of the thought begins to shift. This process demonstrates how defusion can create space between ourselves and our thoughts, making it easier to respond with flexibility and intention instead of getting caught up in the thought's emotional pull.

Goals

- Create distance from distressing thoughts by playing with how they sound and feel
- Reinforce the idea that thoughts are not facts, but constructions made up of words
- Build metacognitive awareness and encourage flexible thinking

Materials

- Blank paper
- Writing utensil
- Translator app (e.g., Google Translate)

Instructions

1. Explain to your client that you'll be playing a translation game. The goal is to take a sticky thought (i.e., one that often gets stuck in their mind) and watch it change form through many different versions. By changing the thought's "language" or form, they can loosen its grip over them.
2. Ask the client to identify a sticky thought—one that pops up frequently and feels hard to shake (e.g., "I'm not good at this," "Nobody wants to be my friend," "I always mess things up").
3. Write this original thought at the top of the paper as the starting point for the translations.
4. Now use different "languages" to translate the thought over and over. You can use real translations (via a translator app or by looking up different languages) or create imagined translations (like speaking in "pirate," "alien," "robot," or even "emoji" form). The more varied the translations, the more flexible the thought becomes. As they complete each translation, have them write down each new version of the thought on the paper.
5. After creating four to six translations, offer some reflection prompts. For example:
    - "How does this thought feel now?"
    - "Does it still feel as powerful or true?"
    - "What's different about it now?"
    - "Is it easier to see it as just words or sounds, instead of an absolute truth?"

Feelings Blocks

Therapeutic Rationale

This activity encourages kids to unstick from thoughts and feelings, brick by brick! Using the interactive metaphor of LEGO bricks, clients can physically interact with their thoughts and feelings and see how some are easier to unstick from than others. This hands-on approach encourages externalization, making abstract experiences more tangible, and also promotes defusion.

Goals

- Physically interact with thoughts or feelings to promote externalization
- Reinforce the idea of separating from sticky thoughts and feelings

Materials

- LEGO bricks
- Masking tape
- Permanent marker

Instructions

1. Before the session, apply masking tape to the side of some of the LEGO bricks for writing labels. This will save time and allow for a smoother flow of the activity. You may want to reserve a few extra pre-taped bricks for later use.
2. Introduce the activity by saying, "Today we are going to think of your thoughts and feelings as LEGO bricks. Before we do that, I want you to take a few minutes to build anything you would like! You can build a castle, a fort, a box, a tower—whatever you want!"
3. Allow the client to build their creation, and during this time, be sure not to comment on what they are creating. Instead, engage in rapport-building and do a check-in.
4. After about 10 minutes, ask the client to stop building. Encourage them to think of thoughts or feelings they have felt stuck on recently—the ones that have been hard to separate from. Have them write these thoughts or emotions on the masking tape on the bricks. This allows you to reuse the bricks in future sessions, either with this client or others.
5. Once they're done, ask them to begin removing the bricks with the writing from their structure. As they do so, encourage them to notice how easy or difficult these blocks are to unstick. Comment that just like our thoughts and feelings, some bricks are easier to unstick than others.
6. Now bring out the remaining unmarked bricks. Ask the client to write down the things they want to be part of their foundation—things like their values, their core memories, their experiences, names of people whom they are close, and so on. Invite them to rebuild their structure with these meaningful bricks.
7. Remind the client that they can do this activity at any time in their mind by visualizing themselves unsticking a brick and replacing it with something that matters most to them.

Skill Practice and Application

Bubble Popping

Therapeutic Rationale

This activity helps clients learn the core ACT concept of defusion by encouraging them to nonjudgmentally name a thought, feeling, or experience and then release it by popping a bubble. The physical act of popping the bubble reinforces the idea that we can observe thoughts and feelings come and go without needing to "fix" or "fight" them. It creates a safe and fun way to practice noticing, labeling, and letting go of inner experiences.

Goals

- Practice defusion by watching thoughts "pop" and pass
- Reinforce the idea that thoughts and feelings are temporary
- Support emotional flexibility through playful, nonjudgmental noticing

Materials

- Bubble wand and bubble solution
- Sheet of bubble wrap
- Permanent marker

Instructions

1. Introduce the activity: "Have you ever noticed how bubbles float around and then pop? They don't last forever. They show up, we see them, and then they're gone. Thoughts and feelings can be the same way. Even big ones! They come floating in, sometimes when we don't expect them, and if we fight them, we get all tangled up. But if we just notice and name them, they can pop and pass. Today we'll practice noticing a thought or feeling, naming it out loud, and then allowing it to *pop*!"

Option 1: Bubble Wand Version (Ideal for Play-Based Sessions)

1. Blow a bubble using the bubble wand.
2. As the bubble floats, invite your client to name a thought, feeling, or experience that the bubble represents (e.g., "That bubble is the thought that I'm not good at school," "This one is my nervousness about recess").
3. Watch the bubble, letting it drift for a second or two through the air.
4. Then *pop* it!
5. Repeat this process for multiple thoughts or feelings. Try silly ones too!

Option 2: Bubble Wrap Version (Great for Sensory Seekers)

1. Use a permanent marker to write or draw one thought or feeling per bubble.
2. Invite your client to name each thought or feeling out loud, and then *pop* it.
3. Watch and listen as it disappears.
4. Repeat as needed, continuing to pop bubbles and let go of thoughts and feelings as they pop.

Haunted House, Haunted Thoughts

Therapeutic Rationale

Anxiety is about the future, be it the immediate future or the distant future. More than that, it is anxiety about an unknown future. At our core, we are afraid that unpredictable outcomes will occur and that we won't be able to handle them. Cognitive defusion is about acknowledging that although we may feel this fear, it is not necessarily an accurate reflection of reality. This exercise helps kids step back from their anxious thoughts by confronting the metaphor of a haunted house, illustrating how fear can be imagined rather than real.

Goals

- Practice cognitive defusion by confronting a metaphorical haunted house
- Recognize that fear doesn't have to define a response

Materials

- Flashlights
- A dark room or space

Instructions

1. Ask your client if they enjoy scary movies, books, or video games. Whether or not they do, ask them what makes something scary. Guide the conversation to the idea that the scariest things are often those we cannot see. Our imaginations are really good at filling in the unseen details with the worst possible outcome. Ask them to recall a time in a scary movie, book, or video game when the unknown added to the fear.
2. Introduce the metaphor of a haunted house: "Imagine you're walking through a haunted house, where everything is dark and you can't see what's ahead. The unknown adds to the fear." Ask your client if they feel comfortable practicing this in your office. If so, turn the lights off and make your office as dark as possible. Ensure safety by removing anything sharp or breakable! Then have your client make their way around the office with no light.
3. After a few minutes, turn the lights back on and debrief. What was that like for them? What did they notice? How did they feel?
4. Repeat the exercise, but this time have them navigate around your dark office with a working flashlight. Afterward, turn the lights back on and debrief again. How did the flashlight change their experience?
5. If you'd like to extend the exercise, swap out their flashlight for a broken one (without telling them). When they try to turn it on and it doesn't work, have them still attempt to navigate the darkened room. Afterward, turn the lights back on and debrief. How was that experience different? What did they notice?

6. After the entire activity, process the experience. What stood out to them? What surprised them? What feelings did they notice? Point out that even though they know your office well, it was still somewhat scary to move through it without light. Ask what insight or wisdom they can take from this experience.
7. Encourage your client to reflect on a time in their life when they felt like they were stumbling around in the dark. What would a metaphorical flashlight look like in that situation? It could be as simple as asking someone for help or reminding themselves that they'll be okay. Perhaps it might look like something else entirely! Regardless, reinforce that feeling anxious does not mean everything has been cast into darkness forever.

Skill Practice and Application

Cartoon Character Voice

Therapeutic Rationale

Humor is a powerful tool in our arsenal as clinicians. When we use humor, we can take the power out of something upsetting or scary and reclaim it for ourselves. Matt often says, "I will never, ever make fun of a client . . . but I will *always* make fun of a thought." This is not the same thing as making fun of a client for *having* the thought. Instead, it means that we collaborate with our clients to help them point out the absurdity (and thus hilarity) of their distorted cognitions as a means of reclaiming their power over their own lives. This intervention helps us accomplish just that.

Goals

- Use humor to enhance psychological flexibility and well-being
- Apply a simple and easy-to-remember strategy for cognitive defusion in everyday life

Materials

- None

Instructions

1. Begin by working with your client to identify a cognitive distortion that is a pain point for them (e.g., "I am ugly," "I am stupid," "I will be alone forever").
2. Then ask them to think of the silliest or most memorable cartoon character voice they can. If they are struggling, you can give them some suggestions, like Mickey Mouse, Patrick from *SpongeBob SquarePants*, or Iago the parrot from *Aladdin*.
3. Explain that you want them to picture that character repeating this distorted thought to them—not once, not twice, but 15 or 20 times!
4. Ask them to close their eyes while they imagine the character saying this. Remind them that you are serious—they shouldn't stop until it has been at least 15 repetitions.
5. Once they've finished, ask what they noticed. Usually, clients will say that the thought doesn't feel as scary, hurtful, or upsetting anymore. In fact, it may even feel a little silly. Prompt them to reflect about why that might be. Help them understand the thought feels silly because they have laughed at it, made fun of it, and decided that they are not going to believe it.
6. Discuss how else the client can use this new skill in their life. Encourage them to practice it for homework, identifying other thoughts to "defuse" with a cartoon voice.

Stop the Sting

Therapeutic Rationale

Metaphors and analogies are therapeutically powerful because they make use of well-known images and ideas. When you can draw on a beloved pop-culture franchise, it can add an extra "umph"! We like to use the Pixar film *Finding Nemo* to help the idea of cognitive defusion really "sink" in. This intervention, which was inspired by Dr. Russ Harris,* helps kids understand that their thoughts and feelings are not necessarily facts, but just passing experiences. Much like Marlin and Dory's adventure through the jellyfish field, they learn to "bounce on top" of overwhelming thoughts and emotions instead of getting tangled in them.

Goals

- Contextualize cognitive defusion in a developmentally appropriate way
- Increase ability to respond flexibly to difficult internal experiences

Materials

- *Jellyfish* template
- Writing utensil
- Crayons, markers, or colored pencils
- Computer with speakers

Instructions

1. Ask your client if they have ever seen the film *Finding Nemo*. If not, give them a brief description of the plot of the film and explain that you would like to watch a short clip together.
2. Search online for "*Finding Nemo* jellyfish scene." Select a clip that begins with Marlin and Dory discussing the dark canyon and ends when Marlin pulls Dory out of the jellyfish field. The clip should be approximately three and a half to four minutes long.
3. Watch the clip with your client. Afterward, explain that our thoughts and feelings can be a lot like the jellyfish in the movie. When we swim directly through the stingers, we can get hurt or upset. But when we bounce on top of the jellyfish, we can stay safe—and sometimes even have fun! Point out how Dory gleefully yells, "Boing, boing, boing!" as she bounces across the jellyfish and turns the situation into a race.
4. Invite the client to reflect on a time when they were able to "bounce on top" of their thoughts and feelings versus a time when they got caught in the "stingers." For both instances, what did it feel like? What thoughts or emotions were they experiencing?
5. Provide your client with the *Jellyfish* template, and ask them to reflect on some "jellyfish" they are dealing with and to label each jellyfish with a specific struggle. As they color and

---

* Russ Harris. (April 20, 2017). *Sushi train metaphor by Dr. Russ Harris* [Video]. YouTube. https://www.youtube.com/watch?v=tzUoXJVl0wo

decorate the sheet, discuss what bouncing on top of the jellyfish would look or feel like, and what getting caught in the stingers would look or feel like.

6. Encourage your client to explain the jellyfish metaphor to their caregivers and take the completed sheet home. Suggest displaying it in a prominent place in their home as a reminder to practice bouncing on top of the jellyfish.

Jellyfish Template

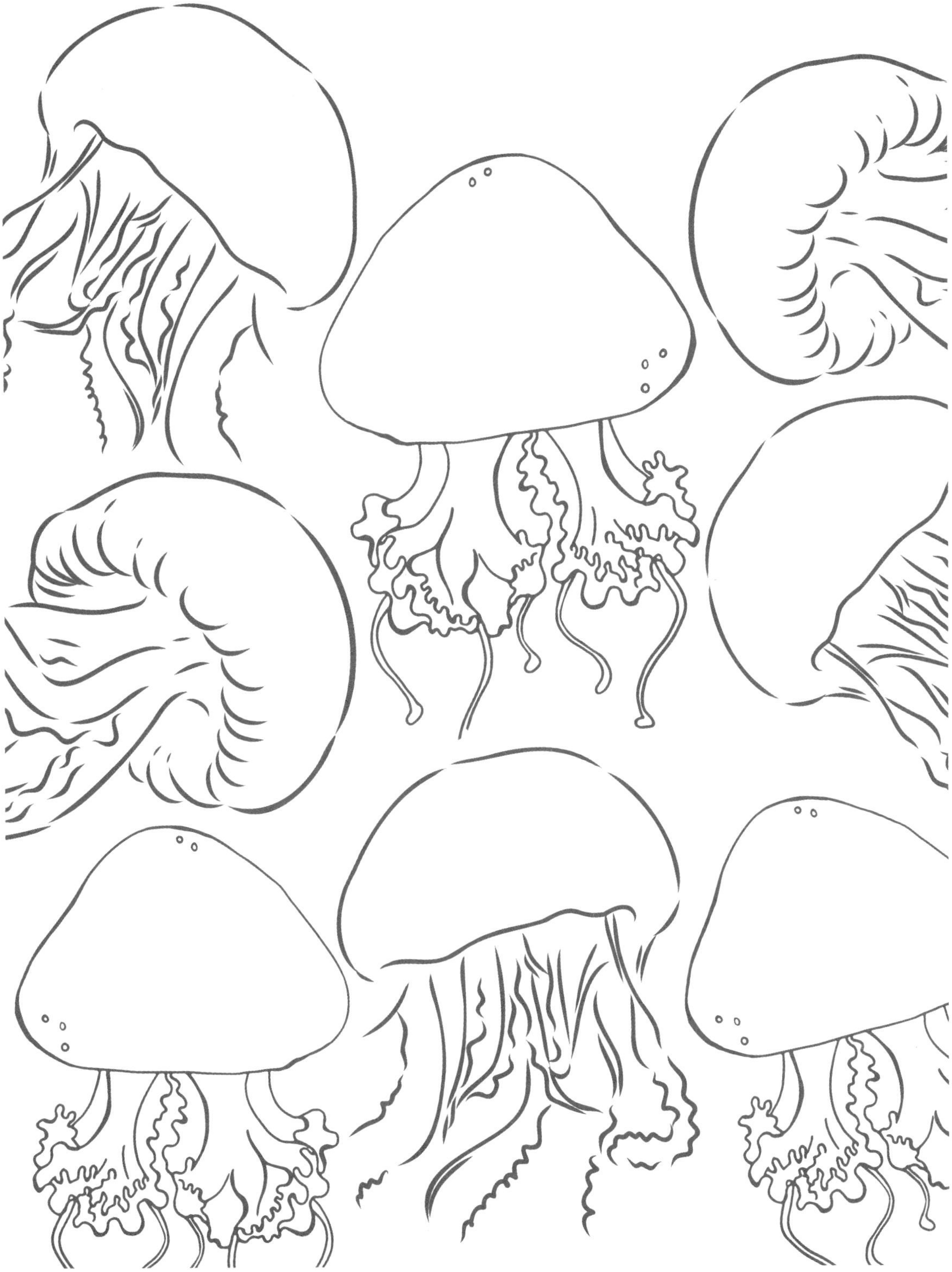

What's in Your Backpack? Part 1

Therapeutic Rationale

Many kids who have experienced trauma carry heavy emotional "loads," but it can be hard to recognize how much weight those thoughts and feelings add to their life. This activity uses the metaphor of a backpack filled with books, where each book represents an overwhelming thought, feeling, or memory that adds to that heavy load. When kids are fused with these experiences, it can feel overwhelming, like a backpack that's too heavy to carry. But by setting aside some books, they can learn to defuse from their past experiences—understanding that these experiences remain a part of their lives but do not have to weigh them down all the time. Note that this activity works best with clients who have at least some level of insight into their emotional experiences and know that they are carrying a lot of "stuff" with them. This is a two-part activity, with part 2 found on page 266 in Section 6: Committed Action.

Goals

- Recognize that all experiences, whether traumatic or not, shape present thoughts, feelings, and behaviors
- Set aside difficult thoughts without ignoring or denying them
- Promote self-compassion regarding the impact of past experiences

Materials

- Backpack
- Variety of books

Instructions

1. Prompt your client to share what "stuff" they are carrying with them, and gently explore what it feels like to move through the world this way. Validate their experience, acknowledging that it must be challenging to carry so much.
2. Emphasize that working through their "stuff" does not mean forgetting it, getting over it, or moving past it. It means learning to carry it in a way that no longer drags them down.
3. Have your client pick up the backpack you have filled with very heavy books. Be careful—you do not want anyone to hurt themselves by lifting something that is too heavy! Ask them to walk around with the backpack and notice what that experience is like for them.
4. Next, have them take out some books and place them carefully on a nearby shelf. They should take out most (but not all) of the books.
5. Ask them to walk around with the lighter backpack. Ask them to reflect on how it feels to carry less weight. Explain that healing from their "stuff" does not mean tossing aside the

books in their backpack. It means choosing which books to set aside somewhere safe. Those books remain accessible when needed but no longer weigh them down.

6. Close the activity by asking your client to consider what this might look like in real life. What feels good or exciting about putting some books aside? What feels scary? Discuss how you work together to set down some of their books, and remind them that you are there to help them carry their load until they are ready to put down some of the heavier items.

Claw Machine

Therapeutic Rationale

Kids often experience difficult thoughts and feelings as urgent or directive. They assume that if a thought appears, they must believe or respond to it right away. This exercise helps children learn that they can notice thoughts and feelings without being controlled by them. The claw machine offers a concrete and playful metaphor for this idea: Thoughts and feelings are always in the machine, but they get to choose which ones they "pick up," which to examine, and which to let go.

Goals

- Differentiate between noticing a thought or feeling and acting on it
- Build cognitive flexibility and emotional awareness
- Let go of unhelpful mental content and shift attention toward values-aligned actions

Materials

- *Claw Machine* template
- Writing utensil
- Crayons, markers, or colored pencils

Instructions

1. Introduce the metaphor to the client: "Today we're going to imagine that your brain is a big claw machine, like the ones at the arcade! Inside the machine are all kinds of thoughts and feelings. Some are helpful, some are silly, some feel angry, and some feel calm. You can notice any of them, but *you* get to choose which ones you want to pick up and hold, and which ones you want to put back down."
2. Explain that just because a thought or feeling shows up, it doesn't mean they have to *do* anything with it. They can pause, look at it, decide if it's helpful, and either hold it or put it back.
3. Invite the client to fill in their claw machine with words or drawings of different thoughts and feelings they've had. Encourage them to include a range of thoughts and feelings—big and small, fun or silly, helpful or unhelpful—to reflect the entirety of their experience (e.g., "No one likes me," "This is fun," "I'm scared," "I can do it").
4. After filling in the machine, offer some reflection prompts. For example:
    - "What thought or feeling is in your claw right now?"
    - "Is it helpful or unhelpful?"
    - "Do you want to hold onto it or put it back for now?"
    - "What thoughts keep jumping into the claw without your permission?"

Claw Machine Template

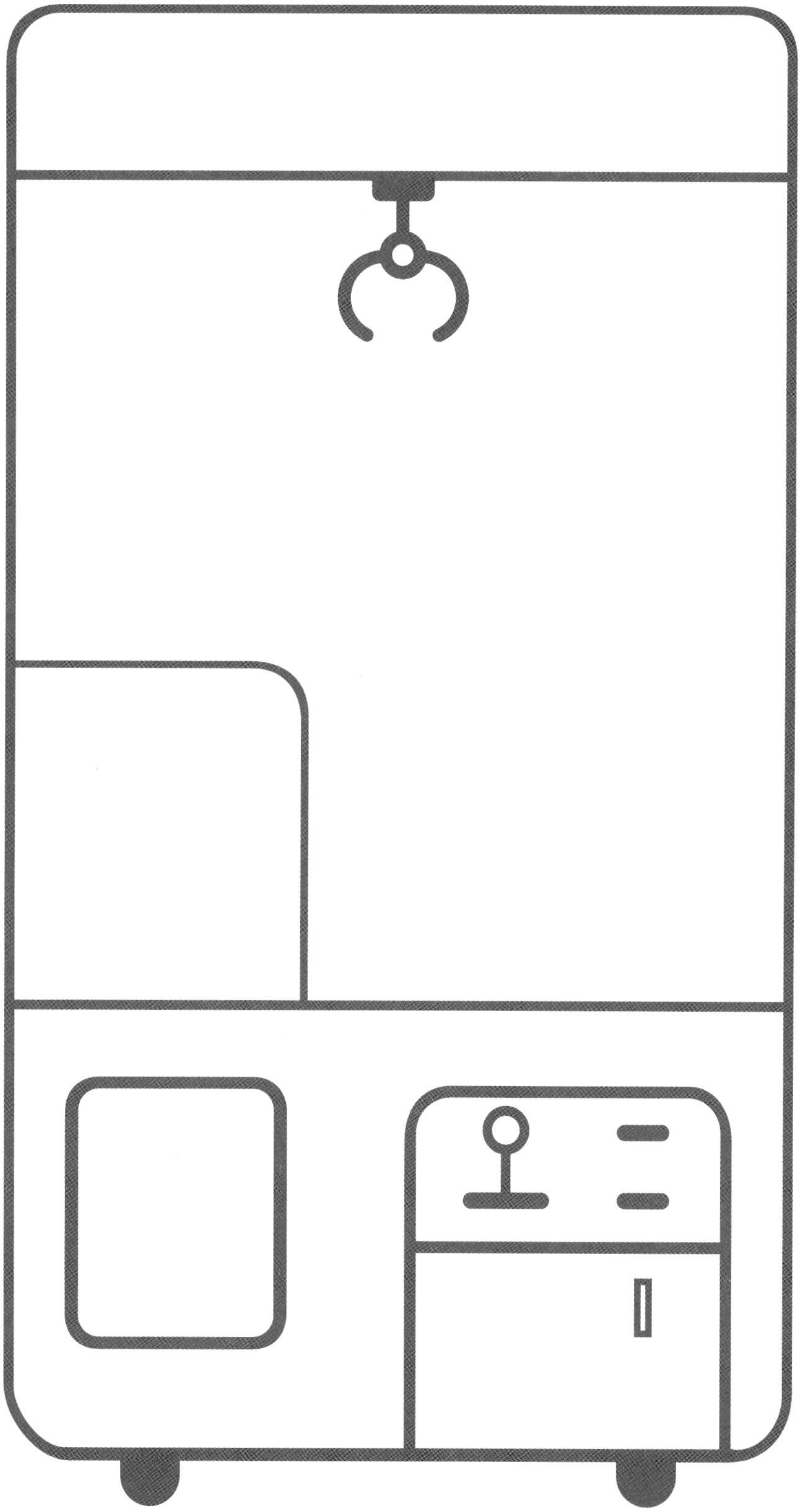

Changing the Channel

Therapeutic Rationale

Many people get fused with their thoughts, believing they define reality. To that end, using the metaphor of a television remote control can be really helpful: Just as watching a television show doesn't make the events on the screen real, noticing a thought doesn't mean it has to control our behaviors. By helping kids identify the "channels" their brain tends to watch—like "The Anxiety Channel" or "The Worry Channel"—and then switch to more helpful channels, they can create distance from difficult thoughts and choose how to respond.

Goals

- Observe experiences without engaging, judging, or being distressed by them
- Shift attention to more helpful internal "channels"

Materials

- *Changing the Channel* template
- Writing utensil

Instructions

1. Ask your client what their favorite TV channels are. Let them go into a bit of depth for a few minutes; this is a fun way to build rapport!
2. Explain that our brains have channels too, like "The Anxiety Channel," "The Depression Channel," or "The Anger Channel."
3. Ask what channels they think they "watch" the most and what thoughts or emotions they experience while watching each channel. Have them list these channels on the *Changing the Channel* template.
4. Explain that just as we can notice when a television show is not enjoyable, we can notice when a current brain channel is not particularly helpful. For example, if we are watching "The Anxiety Channel" and our thoughts are spiraling, it might be helpful to switch to "The Grounding Channel" or "The Mindfulness Channel." Prompt your client to consider what channels they could switch to in those moments, including how they will notice when they are on a less helpful channel. Have them write down these more helpful channels on the template as well.
5. Send your client home with their new channel list, and assign them homework to notice when they are watching an undesired channel and practice changing to a more helpful channel.

Changing the Channel Template

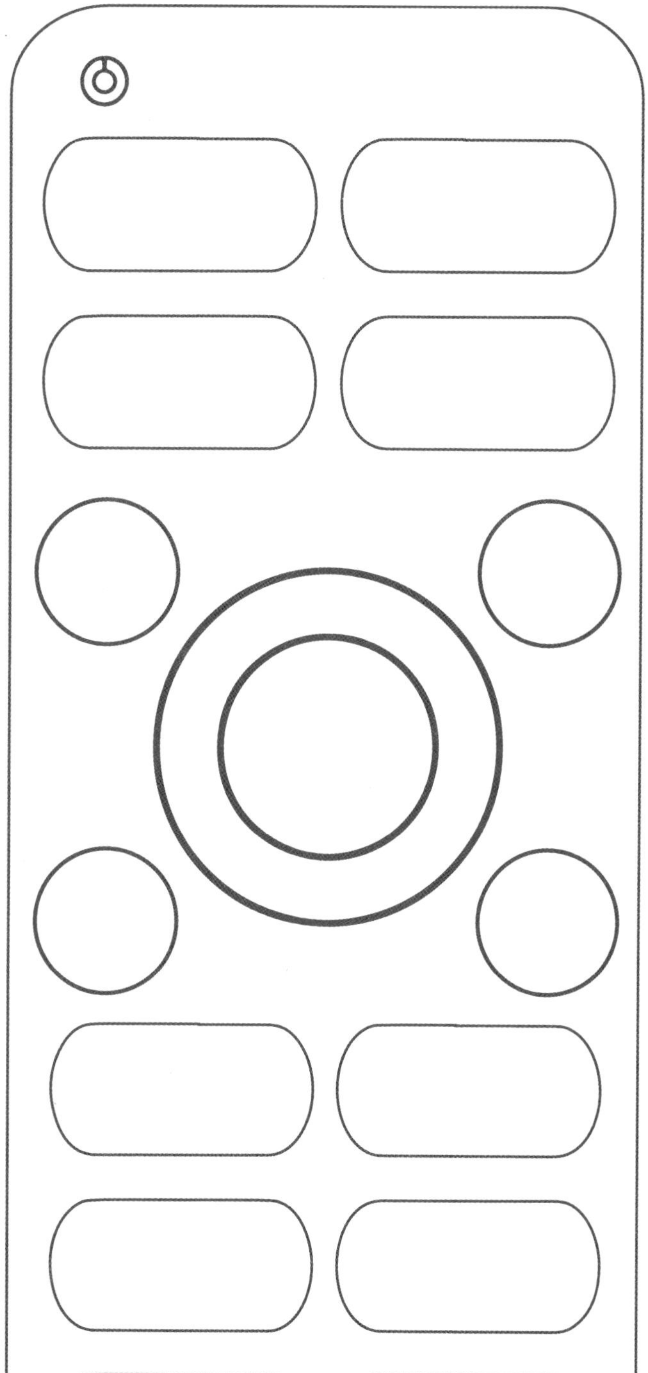

Shoulder Therapist

Therapeutic Rationale

A concept that we borrow from emotionally focused therapy is that therapists can act as temporary surrogate attachment figures. When we are working with kids who have experienced attachment injury or have low self-esteem, they can become fused with unhelpful or self-critical thoughts. In these moments, we can play the role of "shoulder therapist" to help them separate from these thoughts and build up their own internal resources. Most kids are familiar with the concept of a shoulder angel or shoulder devil, as humorously played in films like *The Emperor's New Groove*. This activity encourages clients to develop a "shoulder therapist" as an internal protective voice—a supportive guide that helps them develop secure attachment, self-esteem, and self-efficacy.

Note: It is important to consider your client's cultural and religious background prior to utilizing this intervention because different belief systems may hold angels and devils in different contexts, so you will need to gauge client familiarity and comfortability in session.

Goals

- Repair previous attachment injury or trauma
- Develop internal resources like self-esteem and self-efficacy
- Empower clients to gain trust in their own voice

Materials

- Blank paper
- Crayons, markers, or colored pencils

Instructions

1. Ask your client if they are familiar with the concept of a shoulder angel and shoulder devil. If not, show them a few appropriate cartoon or movie clips for context.
2. Explain that you want them to have a third option: a shoulder therapist! This is a teeny tiny version of you on their shoulder, who encourages and guides them while holding them accountable.
3. Model your shoulder therapist voice for the client by acting out supportive statements they can internalize. Let your humor and personality shine—give examples, play to the cheap seats, and make it fun! Part of the point is to laugh. You want the client to have a very strong impression of "shoulder therapist" you, as this will form the basis of their new internal voice.

4. After modeling, give the client a piece of paper and have them draw "shoulder [*therapist's name*]." Encourage them to capture your voice, facial expression, and key phrases they want to remember. This creates a visual anchor for their internal voice.
5. As an optional expansion, ask the client to recall recent struggles or challenging situations in their life. Ask them to imagine what "shoulder [*therapist's name*]" would have said during those situations.
6. For homework, have your client record at least three instances during the week when they considered what "shoulder [*therapist's name*]" was saying.

Inner Debate Team

Therapeutic Rationale

This activity helps children externalize and observe their thoughts by turning them into characters on an imaginary debate team. By imagining their thoughts, emotions, and experiences as different debaters, they can notice each one's unique qualities: how loud each one is, how strongly it tries to take control, and the arguments it makes. This process allows kids to notice and name their mental events as just thoughts, giving them the opportunity to step back and choose to not listen to unhelpful or distressing thoughts.

Goals

- Develop flexible thinking and self-awareness
- Defuse from unhelpful thoughts and feelings
- Foster a playful, nonjudgmental approach to difficult internal experiences

Materials

- Blank paper
- Writing utensil
- Puppets or stuffed animals (optional)

Instructions

1. Introduce the activity: "Sometimes, it can feel like our thoughts, feelings, and experiences are fighting in our head to be in charge. Sometimes, they can get so loud that it's hard to notice anything else! Today we're not just going to turn the volume down on that inner argument—we're also going to practice choosing which thoughts to pay attention to, just like in a debate where we hear all sides and decide which argument makes the most sense to us."
2. Ask the client to list out each side of the debate in their head:
    a. One side should represent the thoughts, feelings, and experiences that are difficult to unstick from.
    b. The other side should represent the client's coping skills, values, and goals.
3. Have the client come up with an argument for each side. If using puppets or stuffed animals, have them act it out! Ideally, they should come up with arguments for why they *don't* need to listen to the unhelpful side and focus on the helpful side's argument instead.
4. Ask the client to write down key reminders or arguments from the debate that help them remember why it's beneficial to defuse from the unhelpful debaters and engage with the helpful debaters instead.

Train Cars

Therapeutic Rationale

This activity helps kids visualize how they can carry certain thoughts, behaviors, identities, or roles with them like train cars. Some of these "cars" are helpful and connected to their values or goals, while others may slow them down, take up unnecessary space, or even derail them. By externalizing thoughts and choices as train cars, kids can learn to defuse from unhelpful patterns and intentionally decide what to carry with them and what to let go.

Goals

- Develop awareness of thoughts, behaviors, or identities a client carries with them
- Build defusion skills through symbolic detachment
- Connect defusion with values-based direction and choice

Materials

- *Train Cars* template
- Scissors and glue
- Toy train or blocks (optional)
- Prompt list for ideas: emotions, thoughts, behaviors, labels, roles, etc.

Instructions

1. Introduce the activity: "Life is like a train, and we're the conductor. Some of the train cars attached to the engine are helpful, some are just along for the ride, and some are heavy or even slowing us down. But as the conductor, we get to decide which train cars we attach to our engine."
2. Briefly explain how this metaphor ties into defusion: "Sometimes we believe we have to carry every car that shows up—every thought, emotion, or memory. But if we take a step back, look at those thought cars, really notice them, and decide which ones help us move along the track, we can detach the ones that hold us at the station."
3. Using either the *Train Cars* template or toy train cars, encourage the client to label the cars with thoughts, emotions, or memories that frequently show up. You may need to offer some examples, such as "I can't do it," "My sibling is so annoying," or "I love pizza."
4. Once the train cars are ready to go, lay them all out in a line. Ask the client to attach the thoughts that will help them leave the station and to set aside the ones that keep them stuck. Remind them that detaching a car doesn't mean it's gone forever—they can come back to it later and even attach it if they want! But right now, it's just about which cars help them move forward.
5. If using toy trains or blocks, let the child physically attach and detach cars as they explain their choices.
6. You can even act out scenarios where an "unhelpful" car jumps on unexpectedly, asking the client what the conductor does in this scenario.

Train Cars Template

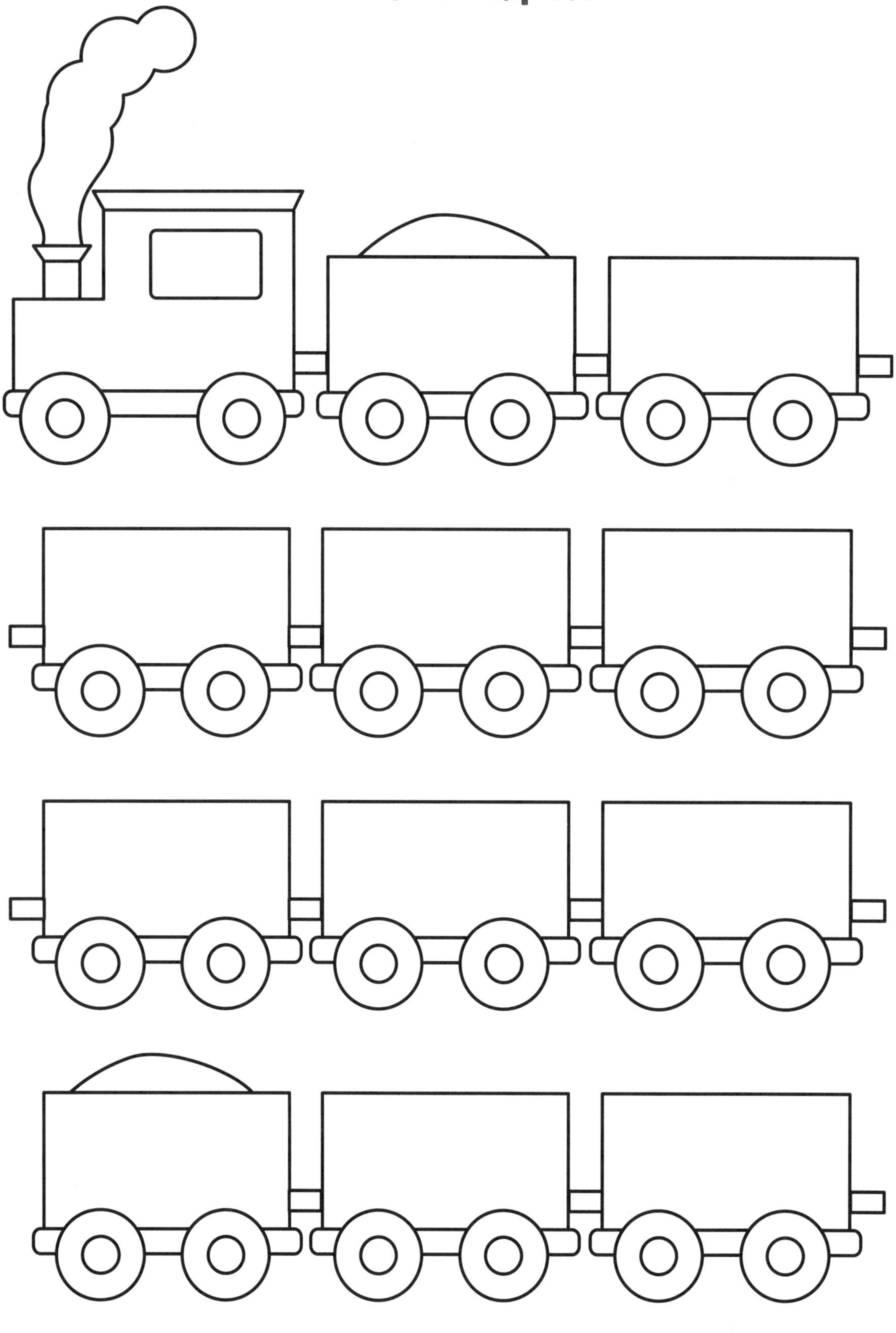

Emotion Monster

Therapeutic Rationale

This hands-on craft activity externalizes emotions and helps kids visualize what it's like when a strong feeling "takes over" and obscures their ability to see clearly. By looking through a fuzzy, cluttered shape with a hole in the center, kids experience how emotions can cloud our perception and make it difficult to stay connected to what matters. As they decorate and explore their "Emotion Monster," they learn to name, notice, and *defuse* from big emotions—not by getting rid of them, but by letting them hang out without taking control.

Goals

- Identify, externalize, and name big emotions
- Introduce the idea that emotions can feel overwhelming without being in charge
- Provide a visual and experiential metaphor for defusion

Materials

- Precut shapes with a hole in the center (cardboard or cardstock works well). Any shape will work as long as there is a hole in the center. Feel free to get creative with squares, stars, or triangles!
- Scissors and glue
- Pipe cleaners or yarn
- Craft items (e.g., googly eyes, feathers, stickers, pom poms)

Instructions

1. Before the session, have a sample Emotion Monster prepared so the client has an example and frame of reference. We also recommend precutting shapes in advance for the client. Cut a large outer shape with a smaller inner circle in the middle, creating a frame to look through. Adjust the size of the shape depending on how big or small you want the monster to be.
2. Introduce the activity: "Sometimes, emotions feel so big that they take over, like a monster sitting right in front of our eyes! When that happens, it can be hard to see clearly or focus on what's important to us. Today we're going to make your very own Emotion Monster to learn what that feels like and stop letting the monster block your view."
3. Give the client the precut shape and invite them to start wrapping it with yarn or pipe cleaners, leaving the middle hole open. As they wrap, ask, "What emotion is your monster made of? What colors or textures feel like that emotion? What's its name (e.g., Worry Whirl, Grumpus, Frustrato, Soggy Doughnut)?"
4. Invite the client to add googly eyes, feathers, pom poms, or stickers. Encourage creativity and playfulness!

5. When they're done, ask them to look through the small center hole. Ask, "Can you see very well? What's it like looking through your Emotion Monster?" Discuss how the monster gets "in the way" when it's big or right up in their face.
6. Then practice taking a step back by having the client hold the Emotion Monster farther away, and ask, "Is the picture clearer now? What happens when you notice your monster without letting it block your view?"

Cloud Watching

Therapeutic Rationale

This activity encourages kids to mindfully observe clouds as a metaphor for thoughts and feelings. Just like clouds shift, break apart, or float by without our control, our thoughts and emotions are always changing. The smaller wisps of clouds naturally drift away from the larger formations, lightening the cloud and changing its shape as it continues on its path. By connecting this natural imagery to internal experiences, kids can practice noticing and defusing from thoughts without judgment or the need to change them.

Goals

- Practice mindful observation using real-world stimuli
- Build tolerance for internal experiences by noticing their impermanence
- Strengthen the ability to let thoughts come and go

Materials

- Safe space to lie down with a view of the sky
- Blanket (optional)

Instructions

1. Introduce the activity: "Have you ever noticed how clouds in the sky constantly change shape, move, and disappear? Just like clouds, our thoughts and emotions come and go. They don't stay forever. They just pass by."
2. Invite the client to find a comfortable place to lie down outside and look at the clouds. If you're inside, they can look out of a window.
3. As the client silently watches the sky, offer gentle prompts as needed:
    - "What shapes do you see? Can you find a cloud that is changing shape?"
    - "Does the cloud changing seem lighter? Smaller? Different?"
    - "Do you notice the edges of the clouds? Are they sharp, soft, or fading?
    - "Can you find a piece of a cloud breaking off and floating away? What happens to the cloud as that part floats off?"
4. Encourage stillness and observation for at least five minutes.
5. Then bring back the experience to their thoughts and emotions: "Just as clouds shift, break apart, and float away, sometimes parts of our thoughts or feelings do too. We don't have to hold on tight to them. Our minds are like the sky—big enough for all thoughts and feelings to come and go. Some are big, some are small. Some float off. Some change. And all of them keep moving."

Sand Eraser

Therapeutic Rationale

We live about an hour from the Jersey Shore, and to clarify, it's nothing like that wild television show! However, most of the kiddos that we work with are very familiar with playing at the beach, so beach-related metaphors often resonate well when discussing the idea of impermanence or letting thoughts and feelings float by. In this activity, we use the metaphor of the beach to help children understand how thoughts and emotions, like sand, come and go with the tide, and ultimately fade away.

Goals

- Illustrate impermanence of thoughts and emotions
- Notice thoughts and emotions with curiosity instead of fear or judgment

Materials

- Sand tray (optional)

Instructions

1. Begin by asking your client if they have ever been to a beach. If so, ask what that was like and encourage them to describe what they noticed about the ocean or sand. Ask if they have ever built a sandcastle (or dug a big hole!) on the beach, only to return the next day to find that the beach looks completely different. Between wind and the waves, the beach is constantly changing.
2. If the client hasn't been to a beach, they can still understand the metaphor of waves coming and going—how waves continuously wash up and carry things away, reshaping the beach over time.
3. Explain that sand at the beach is like our thoughts and emotions. Just like we can use sand to build castles or tunnels, our minds create all sorts of thoughts and feelings—some beautiful, some scary, some strange, and some funny. But the tide eventually washes away the sand, and our thoughts and emotions can also shift or fade over time.
4. If you are using a sand tray, this is a good time to have the client practice writing words or phrases in the sand and then shaking the sand tray to watch it crumble away. This visual reinforces the concept that thoughts and emotions don't last forever.

Security Guard

Therapeutic Rationale

We all possess internal resources and protective factors. No matter how defeated someone may feel, every single human being has at least one thing going for them: They are still alive. To quote an ancient proverb, where there is life, there is hope. An important part of our job as clinicians is often to increase protective factors wherever possible—after all, that is a vital component of building resilience! In this activity, kids will build their own security guard, which can be a fun way to help them internalize important protective factors.

Goals

- Enhance the client's protective factors
- Empower clients to advocate for themselves in both big and small ways

Materials

- *Security Guard* template
- Writing utensil
- Crayons, markers, or colored pencils

Instructions

1. Talk with your client about who is responsible for taking care of them, such as teachers, caregivers, and even themselves. Explain that you want to give them another tool to help them take care of themselves: their very own security guard. (Note that you can replace "security guard" with "knight," "soldier," or another protective archetype as appropriate for the child.)
2. Discuss the ways this security guard can help them feel safe. For example, it may give them affirmations, remind them of the supportive people in their life, or help them manage distressing thoughts and emotions in a healthy way. It is a very versatile guard!
3. Have your client design and color their security guard on the *Security Guard* template. Ask them to consider what they want their guard to look like and what features it should have. Together, create a list of "guard powers," and have the client choose which powers their guard will possess. Remind the client that all the choices are theirs because their guard will live in their heart, not anyone else's.
4. Close the activity by brainstorming ways they can call upon their security guard when they need to. Send them home with their drawing and encourage them to display it in a visible place in their home.

Security Guard Template

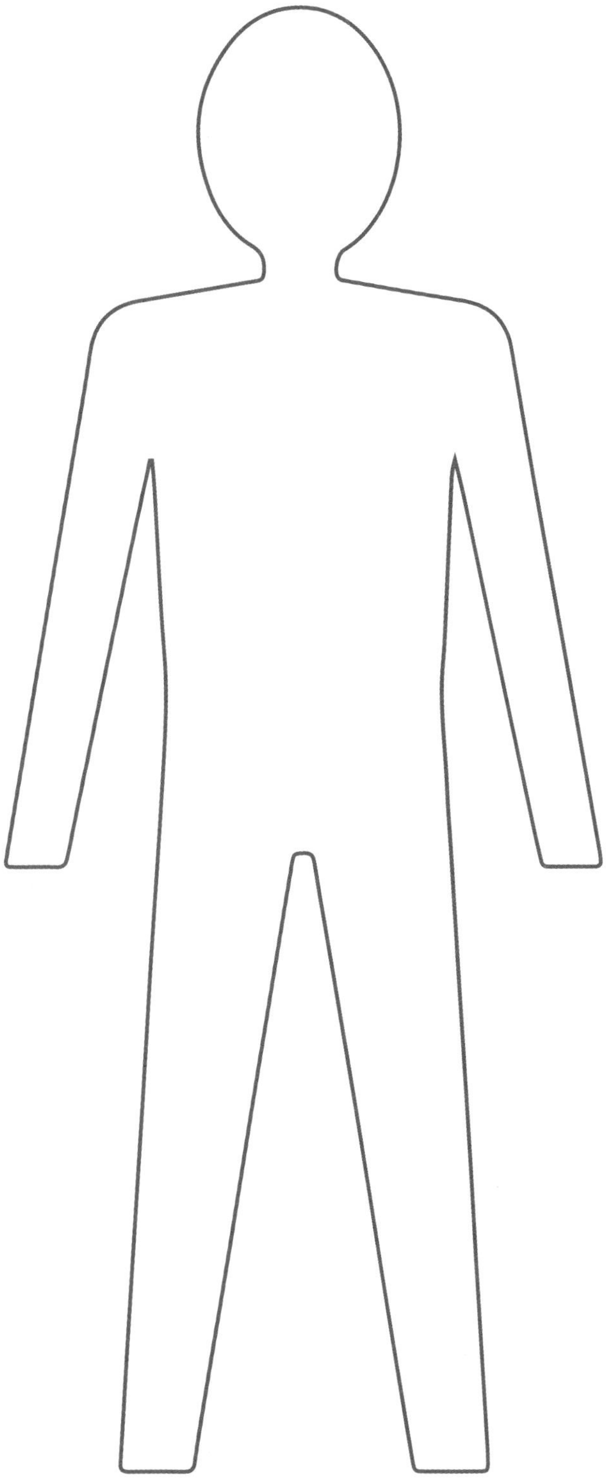

Guard Powers

Roller Coaster Ride

Therapeutic Rationale

Kids tend to have very strong opinions about roller coasters. If you bring up a theme park, most of them will tell you in no uncertain terms whether they absolutely love or hate the experience. Whether they love coasters or avoid them at all costs, they usually have similar reasons for their preference—their stomach drops, it feels scary, they feel like they are out of control, and so on. We cannot think of a more perfect metaphor for life: Whether you love a challenging experience or are terrified by it, it is best to remember that it is just a ride, you are safe, and you'll eventually return to the station, so you may as well just sit back and enjoy the ride.

Goals

- Reframe all-or-nothing thinking
- Gain perspective on the difference between unpleasant and unbearable experiences

Materials

- None

Instructions

1. Begin by asking your client if they have ever been to an amusement park. This question is usually enough to unlock a lot of opinions and memories, most of which will be relevant to the intervention.
2. Ask what they like or dislike about roller coasters in particular. Explain that people who dislike coasters often feel that way because coasters are designed to seem scary, dangerous, or out of control, even though they are designed to be safe.
3. Invite your client to reflect on a time in their life when they felt like they were stuck on a roller coaster they didn't want to be on. Ask what that experience was like and what thoughts and emotions they had at the time. Did they tense up, panic, or try to fight the "ride"?
4. Gently guide the conversation toward the idea that some situations in life feel like being stuck on a roller coaster—we can't get off the ride right away, even if it feels scary or uncomfortable. Explain that in those moments, there are only two options:
    a. We can remain terrified and focus on how terrible the ride feels.
    b. We can sit back, remind ourselves that we are safe, and allow the ride to pass.
5. Ask your client to reflect on a time when they chose option A, and how choosing option B could have changed their experience.
6. Close the activity by brainstorming strategies the client can use to choose option B more often in the future. A helpful reminder may be "You're going to be on the coaster no matter what. Would you rather be terrified the whole time or try to ride it through?"

SECTION 3

Being Present and Mindful

Mindfulness means paying attention, on purpose, to the present moment without judgment. It is about tuning in to what is happening right now, whether that be in our body, thoughts, surroundings, or emotions. The key here is to be curious, not judgmental. That means there are no "good" or "bad" thoughts or emotions; thoughts and emotions are simply "helpful" or "unhelpful."

Why does that matter? Why would we practice noticing the present moment when it sometimes feels overwhelming, boring, hard, or even painful? We do this because being aware of our experience is the first step to being able to choose how to respond to it. Mindfulness is essentially a mental stop sign that encourages us to pause, look both ways, and then go.

As clinicians, it is easy to confuse mindfulness with grounding or relaxation, and while it can certainly be calming, that is not the goal. Mindfulness is a process and not a destination. It helps kids begin to notice what is going on inside and around them with more openness and less reactivity. Through mindfulness, they learn to slow down, name what is going on, and ride the wave of their experiences rather than getting swept away by them.

When talking to kids or families about this concept, it is helpful to explain that mindfulness is like building a muscle. It may feel awkward or even boring at first, but with practice, it becomes a powerful tool for emotional awareness, self-regulation, and intentional choice.

What Is Mindfulness?

Therapeutic Rationale

This activity introduces mindfulness in simple, accessible terms for both kids and their caregivers. It reinforces the idea that mindfulness isn't about clearing your mind or sitting still for hours—it's about noticing what's happening *right now* with openness and curiosity. The activity also models how mindfulness can be woven into daily routines in small, meaningful ways.

Goals

- Define mindfulness in kid- and caregiver-friendly language
- Normalize mindfulness as a flexible, everyday skill

Materials

- A small object from the environment (e.g., raisin, leaf, rock, fidget, piece of fabric)
- A quiet space for three to five minutes of focused attention

Instructions

1. Explain what mindfulness is: "Mindfulness means paying attention to what's happening *right now*, on purpose and without judging it. It's like zooming in on a picture to notice the details so we can better understand the picture as a whole." Explain that mindfulness helps us notice how we are feeling, what we are thinking, and what our body is doing.
2. Help the client practice this by guiding a short check-in. Invite them to get comfortable in their seat, close their eyes if they are okay with that, and take a deep breath. Then ask them to simply notice what the chair feels like against their body, what thoughts are popping in their mind, and what emotions are coming up. Let them know that they do not have to answer out loud. Emphasize that there are no "right" or "wrong" answers, as they are just practicing being present in the moment.
3. For younger clients, or those who struggle with abstract concepts, hand them a small object, such as a raisin, fidget, or rock. Ask them to imagine that they are taking a picture of it with their mind. Now ask them to "zoom in" on this picture and notice the details: the texture of the object, whether it feels rough or smooth, how much space it takes up in their hands, its weight, and so on.
4. Remind the client that whatever they notice is okay. They are simply practicing noticing—sometimes over and over again—until it feels more natural for them to pause and be present. They can practice this same skill in their daily life by pausing before they respond so they can act with greater intention.

Butterfly Hug

Therapeutic Rationale

This activity introduces a simple, body-based strategy for staying present and grounded. By pairing gentle bilateral tapping with calming breath and internal rhythm (e.g., a favorite song), kids learn how mindfulness can engage both the body and mind. This activity also provides a concrete entry point for families to understand that mindfulness isn't just about sitting still—it's an active skill that can be practiced anywhere, anytime.

Goals

- Understand how the body and brain connect through rhythm and breath
- Normalize emotional overwhelm and provide a soothing strategy to manage it
- Lay the foundation for more advanced mindfulness or grounding work (later in the chapter)

Materials

- Gentle background music (optional)

Instructions

1. Introduce the concept by explaining that the Butterfly Hug is a calming way to help the brain and body feel safe. It involves using slow movement and breath to stay in the moment.
2. From here, ask the client to cross their arms over their chest, as if giving themselves a hug. Their fingertips should rest just below the collarbones or on the tops of their shoulders.
3. Instruct the client to start gently tapping one hand at a time—left, right, left, right—like butterfly wings flapping. Encourage a slow, steady rhythm.
4. When first introducing mindfulness as a concept, it may be difficult for some clients to stay focused or calm, and some may also be uncomfortable with silence. In this case, you may pair the tapping with a familiar song to provide an anchor. Invite the client to quietly hum or silently sing a song they enjoy while matching the tapping to the beat of the song.
5. Encourage slow, steady breathing throughout the exercise—in through the nose, out through the mouth—as they continue to gently flap their wings.

Locus of Control

Therapeutic Rationale

As human beings, we are hardwired to want two things: stability and control. We do not like change, and we want to be in charge! However, the world often does not allow us to be in charge of *everything*, and we tend to catastrophize and believe that this means we are in control of *nothing*. This exercise is designed to help kids recognize what they are in control of and to explore additional areas of their life where they can exert more control.

Goals

- Empower kids by highlighting their own autonomy
- Identify and challenge thoughts that contribute to distress
- Notice distress in the present moment and respond with grounding

Materials

- *Locus of Control* worksheet
- Writing utensil

Instructions

1. Ask your client to recall a recent situation that caused them moderate distress. Have them describe what specifically upset them about the situation.
2. Introduce the idea that situations themselves do not automatically cause distress. After all, if the situation were inherently upsetting, then everyone would react the same way. Instead, it is our perceptions, thoughts, and beliefs that create our distress.
3. Continue the conversation: "Human beings want to be in control. We hate when things happen that we cannot control, and that is often what upsets us the most. Let's explore what parts of this situation you are in control of and what parts you wish you could control."
4. Help your client fill out the *Locus of Control* worksheet. In the first column, have them list things they *want* to be in control of regarding the situation. In the second column, have them list what they actually *are* in control of.
5. Once the worksheet is complete, focus on the "want to be in control" column. For each item they listed, work with your client to identify any elements of the response that they may be able to control. Perhaps they cannot control everything, but there is almost always *something* that they can do. For example, they might not be able to change a hurtful comment that someone else made, but they can choose how they respond (e.g., calmly asserting themselves or walking away). If nothing else, they can control their response to the situation—that is something that they are *always* in charge of.
6. Conclude with a conversation about how your client can use this strategy to reduce distress whenever they feel out of control and increase their sense of agency.

Locus of Control Worksheet

Fill in the first column with things you *want* to be in control of, and the second column with things you actually *are* in control of.

What I Want to Be in Control Of	What I Am in Control Of

Breathing Shapes

Therapeutic Rationale

This activity introduces the concept of intentional, mindful breathing in a playful and accessible way. Using familiar shapes as visual and kinesthetic guides helps kids anchor their attention to the present moment, learn breath regulation, and develop a calming routine they can use across environments. This activity lays a concrete foundation for integrating mindfulness into daily life by linking it with something visual, familiar, and fun.

Goals

- Teach controlled breathing using visual cues
- Build present-moment focus in a way that feels playful and accessible
- Normalize the use of breath as a calming strategy in emotionally activating moments

Materials

- *Breathing Shapes* template
- Crayons, markers, or colored pencils (optional)
- Laminated shape cards or window markers for tracing (optional)

Instructions

1. Take a moment to explain how slow, intentional breathing can help calm the mind and body: "One of the best ways to feel calmer and more in control is to use our breath. Breathing slowly and intentionally helps our brain and body work together. And today we're going to use shapes to help us practice!"
2. Have the *Breathing Shapes* template ready to use, draw a few shapes with the client, or encourage them to "trace" the shapes in the air with their finger.
3. As the client traces the shape (on paper or in the air), pair it with the breath:
   a. Trace one side while slowly breathing in through their nose.
   b. Trace the next side while holding the breath.
   c. Trace the next side while slowly exhaling through the mouth.
   d. Trace the next side while holding that exhale.
   e. Repeat the cycle as needed. We suggest using three seconds per side, but find a pace that works best for you and the client.
4. After the activity, offer some reflection prompts. For example:
   - "What did you notice in your body while we did that?"
   - "What was your favorite shape to breathe with?"
   - "When could you use shape breathing to help you—at home, at school, before bedtime, or during sports?"

Breathing Shapes Template

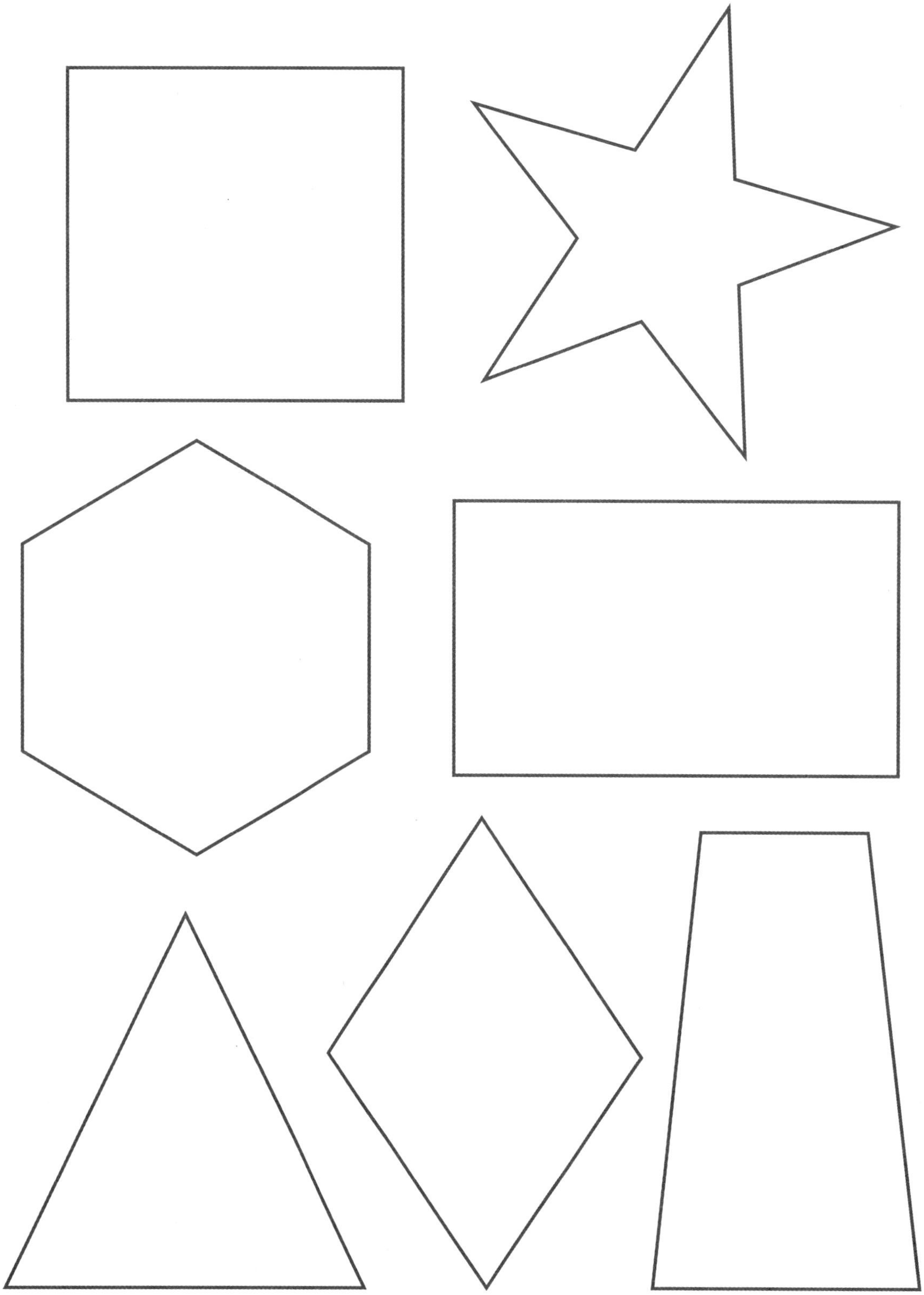

Mirror Breathing

Therapeutic Rationale

The Mirror Game introduces mindfulness and breathwork in a playful, interactive way. By mirroring slow, intentional movements, kids become more aware of their body and breath, which allows them to experience how paying attention to the present moment can promote calmness and relaxation. This activity also provides a fun, social way to practice mindfulness with others.

Goals

- Practice noticing and controlling the breath
- Increase awareness of how the body feels in the present moment

Materials

- None

Instructions

1. Explain to your client that you will be playing a game together called the Mirror Game. The goal is for one person to mirror whatever the other person is doing as closely as possible. To start, you will be the "leader" and your client will be the "reflection."
2. Begin with simple body movements—moving your arms and legs, rolling your neck, shrugging your shoulders, and so forth. Encourage your client to mirror each movement slowly and carefully.
3. Once your client locks in with you, begin to take more exaggerated, deep, slow breaths. If you would like, you can silently count a box breathing pattern in your head, making sure to illustrate clearly when you are holding your breath.
4. Continue the game for as long as feels appropriate. After, ask your client what they noticed about the activity. Was it easy or hard to mirror? How did they feel before versus after? Did their mood change? Hopefully, they should feel calmer and more relaxed now.
5. Switch roles by letting your client be the "leader" while you become the "reflection." Tell them that it is the "person's" job to help calm down the "reflection." Repeat the activity as well as the reflection and processing.
6. Wrap up by discussing how paying attention to the body and breath can help the client feel calm and more in control. Encourage them to practice this game at home with a loved one!

Dark and Stormy Breath

Therapeutic Rationale

Breathing is one of the most natural actions we do. It is literally both the first and last thing we will do in this world. Because breathing is so automatic, we often don't think about it, and trying to focus on it can feel strange or frustrating. Kids might think, "Am I talking shallow, stilted breaths? Am I using my diaphragm? I'm just breathing through my nose and my lungs—I thought that's what I was supposed to do!" To make breathwork more accessible, this activity uses the metaphor of wind moving through the trees on a dark and stormy night to help kids practice mindful, deep breathing.

Goals

- Provide a fun, visual way to guide proper breath technique
- Practice mindful, intentional breathing

Materials

- None

Instructions

1. Begin by inviting your client to tell you, in detail, what makes a "good breath." Expect them to look at you with confusion—that is the point!
2. Explain that they don't need to think about the breath in technical or confusing terms. Instead, ask if they have ever been outside on a windy autumn night, and prompt them to share what it sounded like, felt like, and looked like.
3. Explain that this is the kind of breath you want them to practice taking—breathing as if the wind is moving through the trees on a dark and stormy night:
    a. Inhale slowly as the wind starts swirling in the air.
    b. Briefly hold the breath as the wind moves through the branches.
    c. Exhale slowly as the wind drifts away.
4. Practice breathing in this way together. If they are struggling, suggest they drop their jaw as they breathe both in and out, especially on the inhale. Tell them to just start breathing normally if they begin to feel lightheaded.
5. Optionally, have your client close their eyes and picture a dark and stormy night as they continue breathing. Aim for at least at least 10 to 15 breath cycles.
6. Ask them what they notice after the experience. Hopefully, they will feel more relaxed, particularly in their chest and belly. If you would like, you can combine this activity with a body scan for added relaxation.
7. Finish by brainstorming situations in which your client can use the "dark and stormy night breath" to calm themselves.

Trail Mix

Therapeutic Rationale

Mindful eating exercises can be both enjoyable and helpful—if nothing else, you get to enjoy a tasty snack! This activity is an accessible way for kids to practice mindfulness, as taste tends to be the easiest sensory experience to focus on in the present moment. By paying close attention to the food's flavors, textures, and smells, kids can learn to slow down, notice the details of their experience, and strengthen their present-moment awareness.

Goals

- Practice mindful eating in a fun, engaging way
- Apply mindfulness to everyday activities

Materials

- Various trail mix ingredients (e.g., nuts, granola, raisins, cereal, marshmallows, M&Ms)
- Cups or sandwich baggies

Instructions

1. Have your client select which ingredients they would like to include in their trail mix, place them inside a cup or a baggie, and then mix it up! You can create your own mix alongside them. Be mindful of food allergies.
2. Once they have mixed it up, ask them what they would like to name their creation. The sillier the better.
3. Explain that today you want to practice enjoying a nice snack, but you want to *really* enjoy it. You want to savor each bite, taking time to get every taste out of it that each of you can.
4. Now it is time to eat! Begin eating slowly, encouraging small bites and slow chews, noticing and naming as many flavors and textures as possible.
5. Go back and forth with your client, sharing what each of you are tasting and noticing.
6. As the activity continues, talk about what other sensory details you notice beyond taste: smell, temperature, and sound (e.g., the crunch of a nut or cereal). You can also discuss the idea that there are so many enjoyable and pleasant things that we miss throughout the day when we're not paying attention.
7. Close the activity by brainstorming ways your client can practice mindfully "tasting" or noticing everyday experiences in the coming week.

Grounding vs. Mindfulness

Therapeutic Rationale

When we are feeling overwhelmed, anxious, distracted, or even just disconnected from ourselves, we often hear that we should "be mindful" or "ground ourselves." However, the difference between these two strategies—and when to use each—is rarely explained. This handout helps clarify both! It illuminates what these concepts are, how to use them, and in what situations each is most helpful. You can use it with both kids and their caregivers.

Goals

- Clarify the difference between mindfulness and grounding
- Explain how and when to use each strategy to manage emotions and stay present

Materials

- *Grounding vs. Mindfulness* handout

Instructions

1. Explain mindfulness: "Mindfulness means paying attention to the present moment, on purpose, with curiosity and without judgment. It is like turning on a flashlight in our mind and shining it on whatever we are thinking, doing, or feeling right now without trying to change it. Mindfulness is helpful because it teaches us to slow down and respond rather than react. It helps us observe our thoughts and feelings without getting stuck in them."
2. Explain grounding: "Grounding is a way to bring your brain and body back to the here and now. This is especially helpful when a thought or emotion feels overwhelming or when you are feeling disconnected from yourself and your surroundings. It helps anchor you to the present moment, just like a ship that needs to stay steady in a storm, by reminding you that you are safe at this moment. It reconnects you with your body and surroundings."
3. Introduce the *Grounding vs. Mindfulness* handout and review each column together, highlighting the differences in goal, focus, use, and timing.
4. Optionally, lead the client through a brief mindfulness exercise (e.g., body scan) and a grounding exercise (e.g., 5-4-3-2-1 grounding) to highlight the difference.
5. Ask them to brainstorm real-life situations where they could use mindfulness, grounding, or both.

Grounding vs. Mindfulness Handout

	Mindfulness	Grounding
Goal	Notice and accept what is happening right now	Reconnect with the present and calm down both the mind and body
Focus	Internal (thoughts, feelings, body sensations)	External (senses, environment)
Use	To build awareness of the present and manage emotions	To manage anxiety, flashbacks, dissociation, and emotional overwhelm
Timing	Can be done anytime, anywhere!	Often used in high-stress or challenging moments to bring the mind and body back to the here and now; can also be done as a preventive measure
Example	*Laser Scanner* (see page 105)	*5-4-3-2-1 Grounding* (see page 102)

Skill Practice and Application

5-4-3-2-1 Grounding

Therapeutic Rationale

This activity is a classic grounding strategy that guides kids to focus on the present moment using their five senses. By mindfully noticing what they see, hear, touch, smell, and taste, they can shift their attention away from anxious thoughts or overwhelming feelings and anchor themselves in the here and now. It also builds body awareness and provides a simple way to self-regulate, calm down, and recenter.

Goals

- Shift attention from internal distress to external stimuli
- Strengthen mindfulness and grounding skills
- Encourage "on-the-go" coping tools that kids can use anywhere

Materials

- Textured objects, candles/essential oils, a small snack or drink (optional)

Instructions

1. Introduce the activity: "Sometimes our thoughts or feelings can pull us away from the moment. When that happens, we can use our *senses* to help bring us back. Our eyes, ears, hands, nose, and mouth can all help us notice what's around us right now and bring our mind and body back to the here and now."
2. Guide the client through the activity, prompting them to notice:
    a. Five things they can see
    b. Four things they can touch
    c. Three things they can hear
    d. Two things they can smell
    e. One thing they can taste
3. You can use the optional materials to make the activity more engaging, such as textured objects to touch, candles or essential oils to smell, or a small drink or snack to taste.
4. After completing the activity, ask the client to identify times or places they can use this strategy in their day-to-day life. Encourage them to practice this skill at least once a day. A good place for children and teens to practice is during lunch since there are a lot of sights, sounds, and smells in the school cafeteria.

Alphabet Game

Therapeutic Rationale

This playful and flexible mindfulness activity promotes present-moment awareness by inviting kids to actively search their environment for objects that begin with each letter of the alphabet. It supports attention, cognitive flexibility, and environmental awareness—all foundational elements of being present. Because it's portable and fun, it's also an excellent way to bring mindfulness into everyday routines and family interactions.

Goals

- Promote attention and focus in a fun and developmentally appropriate way
- Provide a portable mindfulness tool
- Encourage family or group connection through shared mindfulness play

Materials

- Stopwatch or timer (optional)

Instructions

1. Introduce the activity: "Sometimes, our minds get busy thinking about the past or worrying about the future. This game helps us practice mindfulness by looking around right now and noticing what's here. Let's go through the alphabet and find something that starts with each letter, starting with A."
2. Choose how to play:
   - **Solo version:** The client works through the alphabet, spotting objects around them.
   - **Partner or group version:** Partners take turns going through the letters.
   - **Timed version:** Set a timer to see how many letters can be completed within a set amount of time.
   - **Family version:** Play in the car, at dinner, or on a walk to encourage shared mindfulness practice.
3. Work through the alphabet with the client, and encourage creativity and problem-solving if the client gets stuck on a letter. For example, you might draw a xylophone for X or turn a horse stuffed animal into a unicorn for U!

Skill Practice and Application

Cozy Corner

Therapeutic Rationale

Creating a cozy corner gives kids a tangible, inviting space to practice mindfulness and emotional regulation at home. By brainstorming the corner together in session, clients gain a sense of ownership and agency, and families are guided to support ongoing use of mindfulness tools at home. This dedicated cozy corner reinforces the idea that being present and calming down is a skill that kids can return to at any time—not just in therapy.

Goals

- Encourage carryover of mindfulness practices into the home environment
- Promote sensory integration using calming, multisensory materials
- Enhance ability to cope with big emotions

Materials

- In session: Blank paper and a writing utensil
- At home: Suggested items include weighted blankets, pillows, fidgets, mandalas, coloring pages, noise-canceling headphones, sound machines, printouts of mindfulness activities

Instructions

1. Introduce the activity to the client and their family: "Today we are going to start planning your cozy corner. This is a special spot just for you where you can take a break, calm your body, be more present, and feel more in control. We are going to make a plan for it today, and you can work on it at home after the session!"
2. Collaboratively brainstorm what the client would like to include in their cozy corner. We recommend discussing it beforehand with caregivers so they can better participate and offer suggestions for items they might already have in the home.
3. If the client would like, they are welcome to draw out their space—encourage them to get involved and get creative!
4. Make sure to discuss why the client wants to include each item in their cozy corner. The *why* is critical so they understand that the purpose of this space is to calm down and recenter rather than engage in high-energy or overly stimulating activities. We recommend limiting the use of screens in this space so the client does not associate screens with being mindful.
5. Encourage caregivers to help set up the space with the client, using their ideas and drawings as a guide. Reinforce that this is the *client's* space and should feel peaceful and welcoming. Remind them it's not a punishment corner—it's a mindfulness retreat.
6. Each time the child uses the cozy corner at home, they can reflect: "What brought me here today? What do I feel now? What will help me feel a little calmer?"

Skill Practice and Application

Laser Scanner

Therapeutic Rationale

Body scan practices help kids develop interoceptive awareness, which is the ability to notice what's happening inside their bodies in the present moment. In this activity, kids will imagine a calming laser moving gently through their body, which strengthens the body-mind connection, promotes relaxation, and grounds attention in the here and now. The playful metaphor of a laser also makes the activity more accessible and engaging for younger clients while serving as a more concrete metaphor for teens as well.

Goals

- Increase mindful awareness of bodily sensations
- Support relaxation and calming through visualization
- Increase tolerance for stillness and present-moment attention

Materials

- None

Instructions

1. Invite your client to lie on their back or sit comfortably in a chair. Explain the activity: "Today you are going to get more in touch with what is going on in your body right now. You are going to picture a laser, but not just any laser—it's a gentle, calming laser that scans your body and brings relaxing feelings with it. As it moves, it helps calm, relax, and check in with each part of you."
2. Use a calm, even-paced voice to guide the client through the scan. This serves as a sample but can be adjusted for clients as needed:

   "Close your eyes if you feel comfortable, or find a spot on the ceiling or wall to look at. Let's take a deep breath in through your nose . . . and out through your mouth. Now imagine a soft, glowing laser light. It can be any color you like—blue, purple, green, or gold. This laser is gentle and calming. It starts scanning at the very top of your head. As it touches your head, your muscles relax.

   Now the laser scans your forehead . . . eyes . . . cheeks . . . and jaw. You might even let your mouth hang open a little.

   Now it moves to your neck . . . your shoulders . . . down your arms . . . and all the way to your fingertips. Feel your arms get heavier as the calm laser moves through. The scanner then travels to your chest . . . and your belly. You might feel your breath moving here. Let it be slow and steady.

Finally, the laser moves down through your hips . . . legs . . . knees . . . ankles . . . and all the way to the bottom of your feet. Let the calm sink in. Your whole body has been scanned safe, calm, and relaxed."

3. End the scan: "Take a deep breath in . . . and out. Wiggle your fingers or toes when you're ready. Then slowly bring your attention back to the room."
4. Remind the client that they can use the laser anytime they need to relax. For clients who struggle to fall asleep or slow their mind down, encourage them to practice it before bed when they are already laying down.

Skill Practice and Application

Warm Ball of Light Body Scan

Therapeutic Rationale

Body scans are simple yet powerful tools that allow us to notice areas of tension throughout our bodies and promote deep relaxation. While body scans will not magically make everything feel okay, it is much easier to feel good when we're not holding onto unnecessary or unnoticed physical tightness. This activity guides kids to practice a body scan using the visual of a warm ball of light that slowly moves through their body, bringing a sense of calm and warmth to each area it touches.

Goals

- Use mindfulness to facilitate relaxation
- Identify consistent areas of physical tightness and tension

Materials

- None

Instructions

1. Explain that you want to practice an exercise that will help your client relax. They will be imagining a warm, gentle ball of light in front of them. Emphasize that the light is not threatening and will not hurt them. It is filled with positivity and goodness.
2. Then guide the client to close or gently lower their eyes as you walk them through the body scan slowly and intentionally. There is zero rush.
3. Begin at the toes: "Allow the ball of light to float into your toes. It moves slowly into each toe. As it does, allow each toe to relax and take in the light. It feels warm and pleasant. You feel each toe slowly unclench. Eventually, the light moves to your feet."
4. Gradually move the light through the body in this order: feet, ankles, lower legs, knees, upper legs, hips, belly, fingers, arms, elbows, shoulders, torso/chest, neck, jaw, nose, and eyebrows. Encourage the client to notice the sensations in each area and allow relaxation to spread.
5. End the scan by saying, "When the ball of light is ready, allow it to float out of the top of your head, taking all of the tension and worry with it. Whenever you are ready, open your eyes."
6. Process the experience with your client. What did they notice? What was the scan like for them? What did they like or dislike? Why? How do they feel now?
7. Brainstorm specific situations where the client might use the ball of light in their daily life (e.g., when they feel upset, before a test, at bedtime).

Nature Walk

Therapeutic Rationale

Nature can be one of our best teachers when it comes to mindfulness. When we slow down and take a walk with intention, we begin to notice more than we ever have before! This activity, which you can do in session or assign for homework, encourages kids to take a walk through an outdoor space with fresh eyes and a willingness to be present, which encourages here-and-now awareness. The goal is not to exercise or get anywhere fast, but to walk with their mind awake and their senses open.

Goals

- Foster present-moment awareness through sensory experiences
- Strengthen the ability to notice thoughts and feelings as the client comes and goes

Materials

- None

Instructions

1. Invite the client to take a slow walk outdoors, whether it's on a trail, around the block, at the park, or even in their backyard. Explain that goal isn't to exercise or rush, but to *notice*. Encourage them to pause often and take their time, letting the environment help them practice being present.
2. Before they begin walking, ask them to take a moment to connect with themselves. What thoughts are popping up? How is their breathing? What do their feet feel like in their shoes? Ask them to pause and notice the weather too—maybe it's a cold day, so they feel the wind against their cheeks. Or maybe the sun is shining brightly and warms their nose.
3. As they begin to walk, remind them that it's normal for their mind to drift at times. That is okay! When that happens, have them gently guide their mind back to the here and now without judgment, anger, or guilt.
4. During the walk, encourage them to notice what they see, hear, and feel, whether it's the crunch of leaves beneath their feet, the chirp of birds in the trees, or the sound of a car driving by. Reinforce that there is no "good" or "bad" when it comes to noticing—there is simply "helpful" or "unhelpful." This applies to any thoughts that arise on the walk as well.
5. As the walk winds down, have them take a moment to reflect. What part of the walk made them feel the calmest? Were there times they felt curious? Was it easy or difficult to stay present? Would they try this again? If so, would they pick the same or a different location next time?

Skill Practice and Application

Mindful First Aid Kit

Therapeutic Rationale

This activity supports kids in building a portable sensory toolkit they can access during moments of dysregulation, anxiety, or disconnection. By grounding through the five senses, the *Mindful First Aid Kit* reinforces present-moment awareness, self-regulation, and independence in managing emotional experiences. Assembling the kit empowers the child to take ownership of their coping strategies and practice mindfulness outside the therapy room.

Goals

- Increase awareness of how sensory input supports emotional regulation
- Encourage self-directed coping and mindfulness strategies
- Build a personalized, portable coping toolkit

Materials

- A small container (e.g., pencil box, makeup bag, reusable pouch)
- Sensory-based items for each sense
- Index card and writing utensil (optional)
- Stickers (optional)

Instructions

1. Help the client brainstorm and collect one or more items for each sense. Ideas include:
   a. **Sight:** Calming image, affirmation card, glitter jar, mood color card, mini kaleidoscope, squishy light-up toy, favorite photo or drawing
   b. **Sound:** Small chime or clicker, noise-reducing earplugs for overwhelming environments
   c. **Touch:** Fidget toy, therapy putty, mini stress ball, smooth stone, soft fabric swatch, textured bracelet
   d. **Smell:** Dried lavender sachet, gum with strong scent, scented squishy toy
   e. **Taste:** Mint, sour candy, gum, lollipop, dried fruit, granola bite (check for allergies)
2. Guide the client to consider which items make them feel safe, calm, or focused (e.g., "What does it feel like to touch this soft fabric?" "What do you notice about the smell of lavender?").
3. Have the client place their personalized selections in the container, and decorate it with stickers or their name.
4. Once the kit is assembled, discuss how and when they might use it. They can write a brief reminder to themselves on an index card (e.g., "When I see my glitter jar, I can take three deep breaths," "When I smell lavender, I remember I am safe") and place it in the container. Reinforce the idea that they might need to use more than one item at a time or a few times to feel present again.

Skill Practice and Application

Journal Prompts

Therapeutic Rationale

In the film *La La Land*, Emma Stone's character tells Ryan Gosling's character, who is a professional jazz musician, that she does not like jazz. He reacts with anger and incredulity: "What does that mean? . . . It's such a blanket statement . . . It's like saying 'I hate animals!'" His point is that some jazz works for some people, and other jazz works for others, but very few people either love or hate all jazz. Journaling is the same way. In our experience, most kids who say, "I don't like journaling" simply haven't found the right approach. Journaling has to be done purposefully; it has to be more than an instruction to write about their day.

Goals

- Empower clients to utilize journaling successfully in their lives
- Provide a variety of purposeful, intentional journal prompts

Materials

- Blank journal
- Writing utensil

Instructions

1. Review the journal prompts provided here and select the ones that are appropriate for your client and their situation. It can be helpful to have them bring the completed prompts to session to debrief and process with them. As a reminder, none of these prompts are for one-time use—the client will benefit the more they practice them!

   Noticing, Identifying, and Regulating Emotions

   - **Emotions weather report:** Your day-to-day emotional state can sometimes feel like the weather. It can be surprising, exciting, or scary. It's daunting to face a blizzard when you are expecting beach weather! Think back on your emotional experience today. If your emotions were the weather, what kind of weather would you be experiencing? Describe it in detail. Are your emotions stormy? Sunny? Overcast? What would help you feel safe and comfortable in this weather?
   - **Body's voice:** If your body could speak about how it feels today, what would it say? How would it rate you as the person responsible for taking care of it?
   - **Emotions at the door:** Notice a particular emotion you're feeling. If this emotion were to come to your house, how would it make itself known? Would it knock politely on the door, ring the doorbell incessantly, or try to break in through a window? What does that feel like?

Noticing and Identifying Thoughts

- **Sticky thought cloud:** Notice a particular "sticky" thought you've been having. If this thought were a cloud, what would it look like? How can you allow the cloud to either rain or float on by so that it is not as scary anymore?
- **Voicing thoughts:** Notice a thought you're having. If this thought had a voice, what would it sound like? Sarcastic, kind, angry, tired? What could you say back to this voice?
- **Protective thoughts:** Notice a fearful or anxious thought. What does your mind predict will happen in this situation? What thought is your mind offering to protect you from this outcome? What might be a more helpful thought instead?

Identifying Values

- **Proud moment:** Think back on a time in your life when you were proud of yourself. What was going on in that moment? What values (e.g., kindness, honesty, courage) were you showing at the time that made you feel proud?
- **Describe yourself:** If you had to describe yourself in 50 words or less, without using your name, how would you do it? What words or qualities come to mind?
- **Role model:** If you could live as a historical or fictional person, who would it be? Which of their qualities made you choose them? How can you bring those qualities into your own life?

Brainstorming Committed Action

- **Important moments:** Think back on your life. What moments or events stand out as especially important or meaningful? What actions did you take that felt good? Why did they feel good? What can you do now to recreate those actions or feelings?
- **Life documentary:** If someone watched a documentary of your life on mute, what would you hope they would notice about you? What would you want them to see you doing?
- **Authentic moment:** Think back to a time in your life when you felt very authentically "you" and at peace with yourself. What were you doing in that moment?
- **One percent closer:** If today you were to move one percent closer to where you want to be, what would you do?

Put It Somewhere Safe

Therapeutic Rationale

Don't run away, cognitive therapists—this is a technique we've borrowed from our friends in the eye movement desensitization and reprocessing (EMDR) community! Much of EMDR work is about noticing and leaving space for our lived somatic experience. In this activity, we'll use a visualization technique from EMDR to help kids compartmentalize difficult or overwhelming emotions or memories in a safe and controlled way. Kids can temporarily store distressing experiences in this "safe space" until they're ready to process them later.

Goals

- Help clients notice and regulate their bodily experiences
- Compartmentalize without engaging in avoidance
- Reinforce clients' ability to maintain cognitive, emotional, and physical safety

Materials

- Crayons, markers, or colored pencils (optional)

Instructions

1. Begin by discussing the difference between avoidance and compartmentalization. Compartmentalization is about keeping something safe until we're ready to handle it, while avoidance is about trying to lock up something away and pretend it doesn't exist.
2. To teach your client about compartmentalization, ask them to think of a place that feels especially secure to them. It can be anything—a desert, a bank vault, an island in the middle of the ocean—any place that feels safe and secure to them.
3. Ask them to close their eyes or soften their gaze, and picture that safe, secure location.
4. Next, ask them to think about an upsetting or scary experience that they want to store safely. Rather than focusing on the specifics of the experience, have them picture it as an abstract image (e.g., a black hole, a ball of fire)—something that represents the experience but is not the experience itself.
5. Ask the client how they'd like to secure this experience in their safe place. They can attach a rope to it and throw it into a bottomless pit, build walls around it, set up guard towers, or surround it with a moat filled with sharks. The sky is the limit! For kids who are not developmentally ready to engage with abstract thought, you can guide them through the activity by drawing or coloring their experience.

6. Have them visualize locking away the experience in this safe place, activating the security measures they've created. When they're done, process the experience with them. What did it feel like before, during, and after the activity?
7. Discuss when it is appropriate to use this technique, making sure that they are not engaging in avoidance by putting *everything* in there.
8. Continue to practice this technique, especially at the end of taxing therapy sessions, if appropriate.

Mission Impossible

Therapeutic Rationale

Younger kids love to pretend and make believe. We can use this to our advantage! In this activity, kids will pretend to be secret agents or spies on a mission, which encourages them to pay attention to their bodies in various environments, especially those that may be distracting or overwhelming. By approaching mindfulness in this fun and imaginative way, kids can connect to the idea of practicing body regulation without it feeling like a chore.

Goals

- Practice body awareness, particularly in public or distracting situations
- Provide a fun metaphor to help kids understand body awareness
- Encourage actions that align with prosocial behavior

Materials

- Materials to make a mask or spy belt (optional)

Instructions

1. Begin by asking your client if they have ever been a secret agent. The more excited and engaged you are, the more likely they will jump into the role!
2. Explain that they will be engaging in "secret missions" throughout the week and reporting the results back to you. Their caregiver will act as their "spymaster" to guide and oversee these missions. You can even help them create a mask or spy belt with "gadgets" for added creativity.
3. Work with the client and their caregiver to create weekly "missions" for them to practice that are fun, developmentally appropriate, and in line with the client's and family's goals. Some potential missions to complete with their caregiver might be:
    - Going into a store and selecting an item off the shelf no more than X times
    - Going in and out of a place without fighting with their sibling
    - Bringing a book or other activity to occupy themselves without being prompted by a caregiver more than X times
4. Have the client and their caregiver write down their missions each week and report back after completing them. How many times did the client successfully complete the mission? What strategies did they use to regulate their body during the mission? Where did they struggle and how can we adjust the mission to facilitate success?
5. Expand or repeat the missions depending on the client's progress. You can also incorporate a token economy system to reward successful mission completion (if you believe it will help and the family has the capacity to follow it consistently).

Security Camera

Therapeutic Rationale

This intervention is particularly useful for kids who struggle with sitting still or managing impulsive behavior. By imagining that they are being watched by a security camera, they can practice self-awareness, monitor their actions, and evaluate whether their behavior is appropriate given their surroundings.

Goals

- Improve insight and awareness
- Decrease impulsive behaviors
- Enhance self-regulation skills

Materials

- None

Instructions

1. Begin by asking your client if they have ever done something without thinking about it, or almost by accident. This could be anything: eating something they weren't supposed to, calling out in class, getting the wiggles, touching something they weren't supposed to, and so on.
2. Acknowledge their experience in nonjudgmental way: "Isn't it funny how we sometimes do things without thinking about them?" Explain that you've also struggled with this and have found it helpful to imagine you're being watched on a "security camera," from which someone important is monitoring your actions. Discuss how in these moments, you ask yourself, "What are they seeing me do right now? How would they feel about what I'm doing? Am I doing what other people are doing around me right now?"
3. Emphasize that the point of the security camera tool is not to feel ashamed or judged. It's to check in with themselves and prevent impulsive behavior from getting out of control. For example, if the security camera shows them standing on their desk while everyone else is quietly reading, this tool prompts them to remember whether standing on their desk moves them closer to or farther away from their goals.
4. Work together to brainstorm ways to remember to use the security camera throughout the day—at school, at home, and out in the world. Caregivers can be helpful partners in reminding them to use it.
5. Assign the security camera exercise as homework, and in subsequent sessions, check in with the client to see how using the security camera influenced their behavior.

Spaghetti Breathing

Therapeutic Rationale

This mindfulness activity introduces intentional breathing in a fun, playful, and relatable way. By connecting breathwork to a vivid and silly image—slurping spaghetti in and blowing it out because it's too hot—kids can more easily understand and remember how to use the breath to regulate their bodies and emotions. This creative imagery engages both body and imagination, promoting calm while making mindfulness feel accessible and enjoyable.

Goals

- Reinforce slow, intentional breathing
- Visualize and embody a calming strategy
- Increase body awareness around tension, breath, and regulation

Materials

- Puppet or yarn (optional)

Instructions

1. Introduce the activity: "Have you ever had spaghetti that was so good you slurped it up really fast, but it was way too hot? We are going to take that same idea to practice mindful breathing. This activity is called *Spaghetti Breathing* because you're going to pretend to slurp the spaghetti in . . . and then blow it out because it's too hot to eat!"
2. Guide the client through the breathing technique, and we encourage you to get silly!
    a. **For the inhale:** "Pretend you're slurping a long noodle up through your mouth . . . Sllllllluuuuuurrrrp!" (Breathe in slowly and deeply through your nose or mouth.)
    b. **For the exhale:** "Now blow on it because it's too hot . . . Ffffffoooooooh!" (Exhale slowly and fully through your mouth.)
3. Repeat this breath cycle several times, encouraging playful exaggeration of slurping and blowing.
4. For younger kids, pair this with a spaghetti puppet or use yarn noodles to make the metaphor more tactile and visual. For older kids, introduce the idea of tension as "boiling water" and breathing as the tool to "cool things down."
5. Encourage the client to revisit this breathing technique during meals, transitions, or stressful events (like tests or appointments).

Three Ring Circus of Awareness

Therapeutic Rationale

Different therapeutic modalities often focus on the past, present, and future. In our experience, life requires us to focus on each of these areas at different times, and when we become too stuck on one area—whether we're dwelling on the past, ignoring the present, or worrying about the future—it prevents us from moving toward our goals. This activity is designed to help kids gain perspective on these time frames in a tangible way. It is most effective for adolescents or older kids with a strong grasp on abstract thought.

Goals

- Encourage mindfulness of the present while working toward future goals
- Offer a framework for clients to consider their life and direction

Materials

- Three hula hoops
- Sticky notes
- Writing utensil

Instructions

1. Ask your client to pretend that they are a time traveler: "If you were a time traveler, where would you go? Would go to the past, stay in the present, or look toward the future?"
2. Explain that, just like a time traveler, their mind can also travel time by focusing on the past, staying in the present, or looking toward the future.
3. Place three hula hoops on the floor in a traffic light pattern. Label the first hoop "past" (bottom), the second hoop "present" (middle), and the third hoop "future" (top). Explain that each hoop represents a different focus area for their mind.
4. Explain that while life requires us to focus on all three areas, we need to make sure not to get too stuck in one ring or another. Ask your client where their mind spends most of its time.
5. Using sticky notes, brainstorm what experiences belong in each ring. Some include:
   a. **Past:** pleasant memories, unpleasant memories, trauma, pain, accomplishments, love
   b. **Present:** steps toward goals, stressors, coping skills, friendships, family, love
   c. **Future:** goals, desires, anxiety, hopes, plans
6. Encourage your client to place sticky notes with specific examples from their life in each ring. It's okay for examples to appear in multiple hoops. For instance, if they experienced the loss of a loved one, they might place a sticky note in all three rings: the past (the loss), the present (the grief), and the future (how it shapes their goals).

7. Ask your client what keeps them stuck in any one particular hoop. Brainstorm strategies to get unstuck.
8. Ask your client what is missing from their present or future hoops that they wish were there. Remind them that while they cannot change the past, they have control over what goes in their present and future hoops. Explore what specific actions they can take to focus on the things they want in these areas. They can also change how they view the past, which might be reflected in the present hoop. For example, they might add a sticky note saying, "I've learned from my mistakes" to focus on what they've gained from past experiences rather than staying stuck in them.

Closing the Tabs

Therapeutic Rationale

In today's fast-paced world, many children (and adults!) feel like their brains are overloaded, like too many internet tabs open at once. This activity helps children visualize their mental clutter and provides a mindful strategy to "close the tabs" in their mind so they can focus on the present.

Goals

- Increase awareness of mental overload and distractibility
- Promote cognitive awareness, attention-shifting, and grounding

Materials

- *Closing the Tabs* template
- Writing utensil

Instructions

1. Introduce the activity: "Have you ever had a lot of tabs open on your computer or tablet? Like a bunch of different games, videos, or homework pages? Sometimes, our brains feel like that too—as if there are lots of tabs open at once! When we have too many things on our minds, it can feel overwhelming and make it hard to focus."
2. Encourage the client to name the "tabs" that are "cluttering their browser." Have them write these down on the *Closing the Tabs* template as they talk it through with you.
3. When they're done, guide them to close the tabs: "Notice each tab that is open on your browser and imagine closing them, one at a time. Take a slow breath in, and as you exhale, gently close the tab. Simply click the X button in your mind. This is goodbye for now, but just like on a computer, you can always reopen that tab later if you need to."
4. After closing a few tabs, ask the client to notice what ones are still open: "What's still on your mind? What's one thing that's still open that you want to focus on right now?" Encourage the client to choose just one tab to focus on and allow the others to remain "closed" for now.
5. Remind the client that they can repeat this activity anytime, anywhere—before bed, during school, or whenever their brain feels too full.

Closing the Tabs Template

Melt the Ice Cube

Therapeutic Rationale

This activity introduces progressive muscle relaxation in a kid-friendly, imaginative way. By pretending to freeze like an ice cube and then slowly "melt" one part of their body at a time, kids learn to intentionally tense and release muscles, promoting relaxation, awareness of physical sensations, and self-regulation.

Goals

- Build somatic awareness and mindful connection to body sensations
- Reduce anxiety, tension, and restlessness in a playful way

Materials

- None

Instructions

1. Introduce the activity: "Today we're going to play a game called *Melt the Ice Cube*. Imagine your whole body has frozen, like you've turned into a solid block of ice! Every muscle is tight and stiff. But now the sun is coming out, and slowly you're going to melt, one part of your body at a time."
2. Start by freezing: "Let's freeze up first. Squeeze everything tight—your fists, toes, legs, arms, and face, like you're a block of ice. Hold onto that frozen feeling for moment."
3. Move to melting: "Now get ready to slowly melt. First, your toes are starting to melt . . . they feel loose and relaxed. Your feet are melting next . . . soft and warm. Now come your legs—they're not stiff anymore, just loose and relaxed. As the melting moves up your body, you feel your belly relaxing. It's warm and soft like sunshine. Your shoulders drop down . . . melting like butter. Your arms and fingers are calm and wiggly. Even your face is melting now—no scrunched-up eyebrows or tight jaw. Just calm. Now your whole body has melted into a puddle of calm! Take a few slow, deep breaths. You're calm, still, and soft."
4. Repeat this activity a few times. We encourage you to be creative! Have the client or yourself "freeze" in different, silly ways like—maybe with a funny face or your hands in a heart shape.
5. At the end of the activity, ask how it felt to freeze and melt. Encourage them to do this anytime their body feels tight or they're feeling anxious or mad. They just need to remember: ice cube . . . then puddle!

Calming Color

Therapeutic Rationale

Color is such a fascinating sensory experience because everyone experiences and reacts to color differently. While one person may feel calm or soothed by a particular color, another may find it overstimulating. This easily accessible grounding activity uses the power of color associations to help kids find calm and peace.

Goals

- Practice grounding and self-regulation
- Promote relaxation through mindful breathing
- Use color as a way to foster peace and relaxation

Materials

- None

Instructions

1. Ask the client what their favorite color is and why. Take a moment to explore the meaning behind the color and whether it has always been their favorite. You can share your own favorite color as well.
2. Next, ask if they've ever noticed that certain colors can evoke certain qualities or emotions. For example, they might equate blue with sadness, red with heat, yellow with warmth, and so on. Discuss how the connections we have with colors can influence our mood.
3. Invite your client to think about what color feels the calmest or most peaceful to them. It does not have to be their favorite color, although it might be!
4. Have your client close their eyes or soften their gaze as they picture that calm color occupying their entire field of vision.
5. While the client continues to visualize this color, instruct them to take slow, deep, and calm breaths—inhaling through the nose and exhaling through the mouth. As they breathe, invite them to visualize the color pulsing gently with each breath—not in a threatening or overstimulating way, but in a calm, safe, and peaceful way.
6. Continue this activity for as long as necessary, allowing for short breaks if appropriate. When they're ready, ask what the experience was like for them. How do they feel now? What do they notice in their body, mind, and heart?
7. Brainstorm situations when your client can use this visualization exercise to ground themselves outside of the therapy room.

Mammalian Diving Reflex

Therapeutic Rationale

Much of mindfulness and physiological regulation involves understanding how our bodies are wired so that we can hijack these processes for our own purposes. One powerful, built-in physiological response is the mammalian diving reflex. All air-breathing vertebrates, including humans, have an automatic reaction to being submerged in water. Our brains are wired to recognize that air is a finite resource, so when we're submerged, our body instinctively lowers our heart rate to preserve oxygen, which triggers a calming response. This activity uses this natural physiological response to our advantage!

Goals

- Leverage the body's natural physiological responses for emotional regulation
- Use the diving reflex to ground and recenter attention

Materials

- Large bowl
- Clean, cool water
- Towels

Instructions

1. Explain that humans have a natural "superpower": the ability to automatically calm down by using nothing more than water!
2. Share how the mammalian diving reflex is triggered when our faces (including our nostrils) are submerged in water, which slows the heart rate and calms the body. In a pinch, covering the face with a cool, damp towel can also trigger the reflex.
3. Together, fill the bowl with clean, cool water, and place it somewhere your client can easily reach with their face. It is better for them to not have them hold the bowl as they submerge their face. Ideally, you should have two bowls of water—one for you and one for your client—so you can demonstrate and guide the process. Do not use ice in the water, and do not add anything to it, like salt, as this may make it unsafe to submerge their face in.
4. Ask your client to take a deep breath, and then have them submerge their face into the water and count slowly in their mind. If desired, you can collaborate with them to create a mantra they can repeat in their head while their face is submerged (e.g., "I can be calm," "I am safe," "This feeling will pass").
5. They should stay submerged only until they start to feel mildly uncomfortable. The goal is to stay under long enough to trigger the calming response but not to the point of gasping for air.
6. Repeat the process a few times.

Skyward Breathing

Therapeutic Rationale

Matt often jokes that he is a trained cognitive therapist who somehow became an attachment and somatic therapist, in spite of his best efforts. This exercise, which we've adapted from EMDR, involves combining breathwork with bilateral movement. It is simple and effective, and can be done almost anywhere, making it a great tool for emotional regulation.

Goals

- Incorporate breathing exercise that incorporates a dash of bilateral action
- Practice emotional regulation via breathwork

Materials

- None

Instructions

1. Ask your client if they have ever played a video game. Most, if not all, kids will likely answer yes.
2. Ask if they've ever engaged in a boss battle. If so, probe further to see if they've ever fought a boss while having their own "health bar" displayed on the screen. If not, briefly explain what a health bar is and how it increases or decreases based on the player's health in the game.
3. Explain that for this exercise, you want them to imagine that there is a vertical "air bar" in their mind instead of a health bar. As they breathe in, the bar rises, and as they breathe out, it falls. Have them picture it in front of them.
4. Challenge your client to practice taking slow, deep, steady breaths while tracking the progress of the bar with their eyes. Their eyes should "push" the bar up and down, guiding it with their gaze. Their head should not move—just their eyes.
5. Wrap up by asking what the experience was like for them. What changes do they notice in their body or mind? Brainstorm when and where they can use this exercise in their daily life.

Mindful Coloring

Therapeutic Rationale

Mindful coloring is more than just filling in a page—it's about slowing down, taking a moment to breathe, and focusing on the present moment. As kids color, they're giving their brains a chance to settle, their thoughts room to flow, and their bodies space to relax. There is no right or wrong way to do this activity! Kids do not have to stay in the lines or use "perfect" colors. It is about noticing and accepting what shows up, both in the coloring and in their minds.

Goals

- Practice mindfulness through creative expression
- Notice thoughts and feelings without judgment or getting stuck

Materials

- Blank paper
- Crayons, markers, or colored pencils
- Coloring pages (optional)

Instructions

1. Hand the client a blank piece of paper and coloring utensils and encourage them to draw mindfully for a few minutes. Invite them to notice how the utensils feel in their hand, what colors they are choosing, and what thoughts are coming up.
2. If they are unsure how or where to start, you can provide them with a coloring page instead.
3. Remind the client that if their mind wanders, they can gently bring their attention back to the coloring without frustration or judgment. In these moments, they can try saying, "I am having the thought that ________, and I am choosing to notice the colors on the page." This way, they can acknowledge the thought while gently bringing their attention back to the activity.
4. After a few minutes, offer some reflection prompts. For example:
    - "What feelings did you notice while coloring?"
    - "Did your body feel different after a few minutes or coloring?"
    - "Were there any thoughts that were especially hard to get unstuck from?"
    - "What did you like or dislike about this experience?"

Mandalas

Therapeutic Rationale

A mandala is a circular design made up of repeating patterns, often used in cultures around the world as a tool for reflection, balance, and meditation. When kids color a mandala, they give their minds a chance to slow down and come back to center. The symmetry of the mandala also provides a structured yet creative outlet for them to focus on the moment. This activity can be calming, empowering, and of course, fun.

Goals

- Support mindfulness without the pressure of needing to come up with an original drawing
- Enhance connection with the present moment

Materials

- *Mandala* template
- Crayons, markers, or colored pencils

Instructions

1. Ask the client to get into a comfortable sitting position and take a few deep, mindful breaths together.
2. Then introduce the activity: "Today we're going to be doing something called mindful coloring. The cool thing about this activity is that there is no right or wrong way to color the mandala. You don't need to worry about staying in the lines perfectly or even how much you get done. It's about taking your time and enjoying the moment as you color."
3. Provide the client with the *Mandala* template and encourage them to color mindfully, noticing that there is no right or wrong way to do so.
4. Whenever thoughts float through the client's mind, remind them to notice and accept these thoughts without judgment, then gently defuse from them and return their attention to the present moment.
5. There are millions of free mandala examples available online, so remind the client that they can continue this activity at home (or even on the go by taking a printout and some coloring materials with them!).

Mandala Template

Bubble Blowing

Therapeutic Rationale

In a world full of distractions (like a field full of bubbles!), kids often feel pulled in many directions. This activity uses the natural appeal of bubbles to enhance focused attention and mindful observation. It teaches kids to intentionally direct their focus toward one bubble at a time while letting go of competing stimuli.

Goals

- Develop selective attention and mindful focus
- Increase tolerance for waiting and observing
- Anchor attention during emotionally charged or overstimulating moments

Materials

- Bubble wand and bubble solution

Instructions

1. Ask the client if they've ever tried to follow just *one* bubble in a big group of bubbles, and explain that today they're going to practice doing just that. They're going to slow things down, choose one bubble, and stay with it, no matter what the other bubbles are doing.
2. Create a field of bubbles by blowing a large number of bubbles into the air, allowing the client to watch and interact with all the bubbles for a moment.
3. Blow a new batch of bubbles, but this time, tell the client to choose just *one* to follow with their eyes. Encourage them to pretend that the rest of the bubbles aren't even there. Have them track that one bubble until it pops or touches the ground. They should observe the bubble closely—noticing what it looks like, how it floats, how it moves, whether it drifts fast or slow, and how long it takes to pop.
4. Do a few rounds of this exercise, blowing a new field of bubbles as needed. Encourage the client to choose a different bubble should their chosen one pop.

Simon Mindfully Says

Therapeutic Rationale

Simon Says is a game that almost everyone understands how to play. We use it with little kids to develop body awareness, improve motor skills, and enhance coordination—and because it's fun! This adapted version of the activity introduces mindfulness into the game by encouraging kids to focus on their bodily sensations and be more attuned to how their body responds to various moments. It can be adapted for kids of all ages to practice exploring what feels good in the body.

Goals

- Promote development of body awareness
- Mindfully explore pleasant and unpleasant sensations in the body

Materials

- None

Instructions

1. Begin by playfully challenging your client to a game of Simon Says, but with a twist. Explain that for this version, you want them to practice noticing different sensations in their body. If you feel that more guidance is necessary, have them stick to noticing sensations in one specific part of their body for the entire experience (e.g., "No matter what Simon says, always pay attention to what it feels like in your tummy").
2. Lead your client through a series of stretches and movements via the game (e.g., "Simon says stretch your arms up to the sky"). They should stretch high, stretch low, and move in different directions based on your directions, making use of their entire personal space.
3. After each prompt, pause to ask them what they are noticing in that body part. For example, "What do you notice in your body when you're stretching up high? Is it a pleasant or unpleasant feeling?"
4. Continue the exercise, focusing on and noticing different parts of their body. If you'd like, you can have them take on the role of Simon and instruct you to notice parts of your body. When they guide you, have them explore what *you* are noticing in your body. This can be a very fruitful topic of conversation!
5. Conclude the game by asking them to reflect on what the experience was like. Was it pleasant or uncomfortable? What made it feel that way? For homework, you can have them lead their loved ones through the exercise at home, making sure to include the mindfulness components.

Cloud Meditation

Therapeutic Rationale

Meditation is like giving your brain a warm hug. It helps the mind and body slow down and feel safe, calm, and clear. This guided meditation, which asks kids to imagine that they are floating on a soft cloud, introduces them to the calming effects of meditation in an engaging and accessible way. The purpose is to show how meditation can calm the brain and body, encouraging them to return to the present.

Goals

- Introduce the idea of meditation while promoting calm, intention-filled thinking
- Increase body awareness and present-moment focus

Materials

- None

Instructions

1. Invite the client to find a comfortable position either sitting or lying down. Explain that it can sometimes be tricky to know *what* to focus on when practicing mindfulness and that meditation can help by giving their brain something to focus on while still being present.
2. Let the client know that today they'll be going on a peaceful cloud adventure in their mind. All they have to do is listen to your voice and breathe gently.
3. Invite the client to close their eyes or gently soften their gaze. Then begin the meditation, adapting the script to fit the needs and developmental age of your client:

   "Take a deep breath in through your nose . . . and slowly, slowly, let it out through your mouth. Feel your body becoming still and calm.

   Now imagine a big, fluffy cloud floating down from the blue sky. It's soft and squishy, like a big piece of cotton candy.

   This cloud gently scoops you up and cradles you like a cozy hug. You feel light and safe as it gently carries you above the ground.

   As you float on the cloud, take a moment to notice the world around you. Maybe you see snowy mountains in the distance or a gurgling river below. You hear birds singing and smell flowers in the field.

   Take it all in. You again breathe slowly in through your nose . . . and out through your mouth . . . feeling your shoulders relax further into the cloud.

The cloud floats wherever you want it to go. Maybe it floats you to your favorite beach, where you hear the waves as they wash against the sand. Maybe it takes you on a ski trip and the cold nips at your ears.

Now the cloud is slowly floating back down, bringing you back to the ground. As you get closer to landing, begin to bring gentle movement back to your body. Slowly wiggle your fingers and toes. Roll your shoulders and head.

As you land, you take one more deep breath in . . . and out.

When you're ready, open your eyes. You're back, but the cloud is always there, ready to bring calm whenever you need it."

Magical Forest Meditation

Therapeutic Rationale

Meditation helps us slow down, breathe, and pay attention to what's happening inside and around us. It's like going on a little trip in our imagination to help our bodies and brains feel calm and clear. In this meditation, kids will take a peaceful walk through a magical forest using their imagination.

Goals

- Encourage sensory awareness and imaginative calm
- Strengthen emotional regulation through breath and visualization

Materials

- None

Instructions

1. Invite the client to find a comfortable position either sitting or lying down. Explain that it can sometimes be tricky to know *what* to focus on when practicing mindfulness and that meditation can help by giving their brain something to focus on while still being present.
2. Let the client know that today they'll be going to go on a forest walk in their mind. All they have to do is listen to your voice and breathe gently.
3. Invite the client to close their eyes or gently soften their gaze. Then begin the meditation, adapting the script to fit the needs and developmental age of your client:

    "Take a deep breath in through your nose . . . and out through your mouth. Feel your body becoming still, like the quiet earth beneath you.

    Now imagine you're standing at the edge of a beautiful forest. You see tall trees, soft moss, and golden sunlight peeking through the branches.

    You take a step into the forest. Your feet feel the soft ground . . . maybe it's a little squishy, or maybe it's covered in crunchy leaves.

    As you walk slowly and calmly, you hear the sound of birds singing above, the breeze blowing gently through the trees, and a stream burbling nearby. Maybe you even hear a fish jump in the water.

    Take a breath in through your nose . . . What does the forest smell like? Fresh? Earthy? Sweet?

    As you continue walking, you see a tiny animal watching you from behind a tree. Maybe it's a squirrel, a deer, or even a magical creature. You smile at it and keep walking.

    The sunlight is warm on your face, and the shade is cool on your arms. You feel safe. Calm. Steady.

If a thought or worry pops up in your head, you can imagine gently placing it in a leaf and watching it float away down a stream.

Breathe in . . . and out.

Keep walking a little more . . . taking your time . . . just noticing.

After a while, you find a comfortable rock or stump and take a seat. You close your eyes and just listen to the peaceful sounds of the forest.

Breathe in the peace.

When you're ready, imagine gently standing up and walking back toward the forest's edge. You step out of the woods and into the light.

Wiggle your fingers . . . wiggle your toes . . . Take one more deep breath in . . . and let it go.

When you're ready, you can open your eyes. You're back, but the forest is always waiting in your imagination."

SECTION 4

Self-as-Context

On the television show *Ted Lasso*, one of the characters, Jamie Tartt, is asked whether he would prefer to be a lion or a panda. His response? "Coach, I'm me. Why would I want to be anything else?"

Jamie raises a good point. Why would any of us want to be anything other than our perfectly wonderful selves? We are all the most skilled people in the entire universe at being *us*. That is a profound and marvelous truth, and a reminder that our existence is a gift. Viewing your life through the context of who you are as a person is the only way that life makes any sense. If you are able to identify what is important and meaningful to you, you can engage in the pursuit of these elements for the rest of your life.

This is often easier said than done. We feel so much pressure, both internal and external, to be or say or do certain things. We learn that if we do not measure up to the standards of others, then we cannot ever be enough. Using and living in the idea of self-as-context is a fundamental rejection of that idea. Self-as-context is the notion that we can step back from our thoughts, feelings, and experiences and observe them without being defined by them. It's about seeing ourselves as "the observer"—not as the thoughts or emotions we're experiencing. When we live from this perspective, the only person who can ever define whether we do enough, whether we *are* enough, is us. Kids can find this concept terrifying. It is scary to be your own boss! Once you are able to help them internalize this concept and believe it to their core, the sky will truly be their only limit.

What Is Self-as-Context?

Therapeutic Rationale

Introducing the concept of self-as-context to caregivers is a foundational part of supporting kids in therapy. This is an abstract and challenging concept for most people, let alone kids! By getting the child's caregiver involved in the process, you can create a shared language that supports the generalization of skills and ideas across settings. This intervention explains what self-of-context is for kids and their grown-ups, highlighting the idea that we are not defined by our thoughts or emotions—we are simply the "observer" of those experiences.

Goals

- Provide psychoeducation to families regarding self-as-context
- Generalize skills and ideas across context through the shared language

Materials

- None

Instructions

1. Explain that self-as-context is one of the six core processes in ACT and is also one of the most abstract to explain. But at its heart, it's about helping clients recognize that they are more than their thoughts, feelings, or roles.
2. Discuss how we often spend so much time focusing on what we think or feel (e.g., "I'm sad," "I'm not good at this," "I don't belong") that we start to believe those things define us. Self-as-context teaches us that we are not those thoughts or feelings. Instead, we are the *observer* of those inner experiences. This is the part of us that is always there, noticing what's happening inside and outside of us, without being swallowed up by it. For example, instead of saying, "I'm not good at this," self-as-context would encourage us to say, "I'm having the thought that I'm not good at this."
3. Explain that the idea of self-as-context can be a powerful shift for kids who feel consumed by anxiety, sadness, or frustration. Rather than teaching them to erase or deny those feelings, we help them observe and hold space for those thoughts without letting them take over.
4. Encourage caregivers to practice this concept with kids in everyday situations. For example, if their child feels anxious about an upcoming math test, they can remind them that thoughts like "I'm going to mess up" are just thoughts, not facts. Similarly, if their child is feeling angry, the caregiver can guide them to notice "I'm feeling mad right now" rather than "I *am* mad."

"I" Statements

Therapeutic Rationale

At first glance, it might seem curious that a book based on ACT includes a section on about communication. Isn't that for systems therapists or DBT clinicians? Not exactly. Here's the thing: In ACT, we take a holistic approach by treating people as *people*, not as problems. With that in mind, we would be remiss if we did not include some of the basics of effective communication. "I" statements promote effective communication by helping kids express their feelings without blaming or accusing others. By focusing on their own experience (e.g., "I feel upset" versus "You made me mad"), they can communicate more clearly and reduce defensiveness. It also facilitates self-as-context by allowing them to separate their emotions from their identity (e.g., "I am mad" versus "I feel mad"), leading to more thoughtful conversations.

Goals

- Use "I" statements to communicate more effectively
- Express thoughts and feelings without blame or judgment

Materials

- None

Instructions

1. Ask your client if they have ever heard of an "I" statement. You can do this in a humorous way if you'd like—we know one clinician who keeps a big, gooey fake eyeball in their office for this exact purpose!
2. Explain that an "I" statement is a way of expressing our thoughts, feeling, or needs without blaming or accusing anyone. An "I" statement is simply a way to share information.
3. Explain that there are different kinds of "I" statements, but they all have the same basic structure: They begin with "I" and then a verb. For example:
    - I thought . . .
    - I feel/felt . . .
    - I want/wanted . . .
    - I like/didn't like . . .
4. Practice creating "I" statements with your client, making sure to emphasize that simply using the word "I" doesn't make it an "I" statement. For example, "I was really upset because you are a big jerk!" is not an "I" statement—it's an accusation. The point is to communicate, not insult or blame.
5. Brainstorm situations where they think using an "I" statement may be helpful, and have them practice creating and using these statements for homework.

The Iceberg of Me

Therapeutic Rationale

This activity helps kids explore the difference between their external behaviors (what others see) and their internal experiences (what's really going on inside). By connecting this to the idea of self-as-context, kids can understand that while they may feel or act in certain ways, they are *not defined* by those feelings or behaviors. They are the "noticer" of both—and by noticing, they are better able to engage with their thoughts and emotions and choose how to best respond.

Goals

- Build awareness of underlying thoughts and feelings that drive behaviors
- Separate the *self* from their experiences (thoughts, feelings, actions)
- Strengthen emotional insight and create language for complex emotions

Materials

- *Iceberg* template
- Writing utensil

Instructions

1. Introduce the *Iceberg* template to the child. Point to the small section of the iceberg sticking out above the water and ask, "What are some things people can *see* about you?" Examples might include "I get quiet in class," "I smile a lot," "I get mad and stomp off," or "I help others when they're sad."
2. Have the client write or draw these external behaviors in the top portion of the template.
3. Next, point to the much larger part of the iceberg beneath the waterline and ask, "What are some thoughts or feelings that might be under the surface?" Examples might include "I feel scared that I'll mess up," "I want people to like me," "I feel left out," or "I wish someone would ask me what's wrong."
4. Have the client write or draw these internal experiences in the bottom portion.
5. Remind the client that this activity is about noticing, not judging. These are just things they've *noticed* about themselves—not things that define who they are: "You are *more* than just what people see. You have thoughts, feelings, hopes, and fears. And you can notice all of them without being trapped by them. That part of you that sees the whole iceberg, that's the *real you*."
6. You can use this activity with individual emotions as well. For example, you could discuss how anger often masks other emotions like embarrassment, guilt, or loneliness. This helps clients connect with their emotions on a deeper level and recognize that they are often multilayered.

Iceberg Template

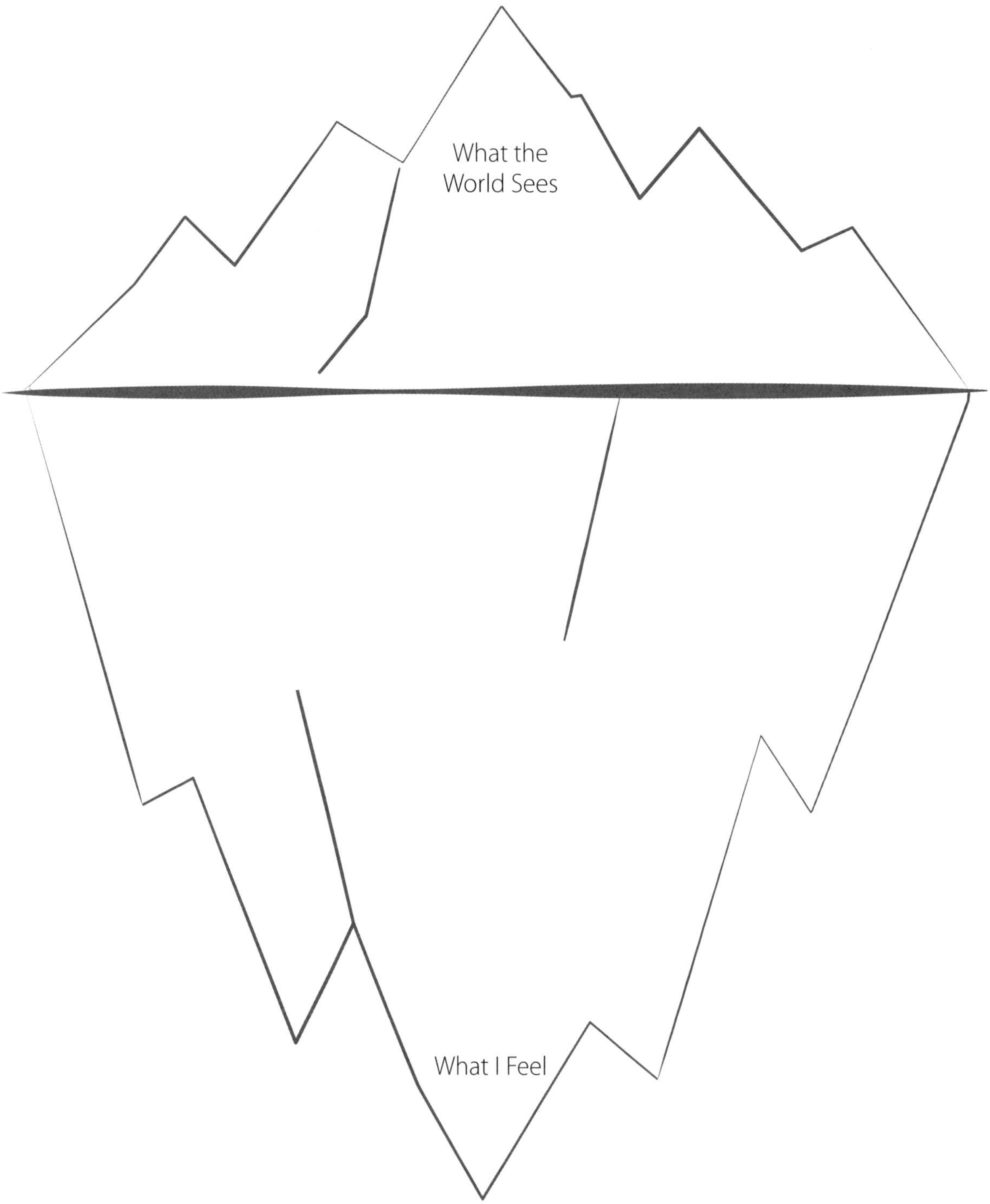

I Want It, I Need It

Therapeutic Rationale

It is safe to say that we've all had clients who struggle with all-or-nothing thinking—children and adolescents often have an especially difficult time with nuance and patience! For kids who struggle with impulsivity or constantly want the latest thing, it can be difficult to distinguish between *wanting* something and *needing* something. This activity helps kids make that distinction. It also teaches them that while their needs should always be met, there are more productive ways to get more of what they want. This helps lay the groundwork for self-as-context by helping them observe their desires without letting it consume their identity.

Goals

- Distinguish wants from needs
- Facilitate healthy communication regarding wants, needs, and household contributions

Materials

- *I Want It, I Need It* worksheet
- Writing utensil

Instructions

1. Ask the client to distinguish between a want and a need. Explain that a need is something that we can't live without, such as food, water, clothing, shelter, love, and education, while a want is something we desire but can live without.
2. Help the client list examples from their own life using the *I Want It, I Need It* worksheet, separating "I Want" items (e.g., a new toy or video game) from "I Need" items (e.g., food at every meal, new clothing when they outgrow their current size).
3. Ask the client how their *needs* are being met, acknowledging that caregivers and other grown-ups typically provide these basic necessities. This will probably be a short conversation, as it is usually a legal requirement that children get their needs met.
4. Next, discuss how the client can increase the chances of getting their *wants* met. Explain that the more they contribute to the household (e.g., doing chores, following rules), the more likely they are to receive their wants.
5. Use the *I Want It, I Need It* worksheet to have the client list tasks they can help with in the "I Can Do" column. This might include doing homework, walking the dog, or taking out the trash. Be sure to emphasize that the exchange is not always a one-to-one equivalent. For example, completing two tasks doesn't guarantee getting two wants.
6. If they feel like their "I Can Do" list outweighs their wants being met, that can prompt a conversation with the client and their caregiver to ensure fairness and balance.

7. As an optional extension, have the caregiver fill out the worksheet from their perspective, listing what they want, need, and do for the family. Sharing this with the client in an informative (and non-shaming) way can lead to greater understanding and empathy between both parties.

I Want It, I Need It Worksheet

Write down things you want (e.g., a new toy or video game) in the "I Want" column, and things you need (e.g., food, water, clothes) in the "I Need" column. In the "I Can Do" column, think about what you can do for your household to earn more of what you want (e.g., walk the dog, take out the trash).

I Want	I Need	I Can Do

What Goes on Your Name Tag?

Therapeutic Rationale

Most people will swear that they know themselves intimately . . . until they are asked to share *what* it is that they know about themselves. Kids in particular often struggle to explicitly identify who they are or what descriptors resonate with them. They know who they are in the sense that they have spent literally every second of their lives with their own thoughts and experiences, but that closeness can make it difficult to see the forest for the trees. This activity is designed to help them step back and explore who they are.

Goals

- Promote self-awareness and self-concept
- Encourage reflection on personal identity

Materials

- Name tags
- Writing utensil
- Crayons, markers, or colored pencils

Instructions

1. Ask your client to share their favorite quality about themselves. Are they kind? Smart? Funny? There are so many wonderful qualities that they may embody! Ask how they decided which quality to pick.
2. Take a moment to process that experience with your client. What was it like to think about themselves that way? Was it easy or hard? Did it feel awkward or embarrassing? If so, why?
3. Explain that you want to get to know them better and help others see how awesome they are—and to do that, you're going to use name tags.
4. Together, brainstorm adjectives that describe your client. Gently ask evidence: How do they know this is true? (The point of asking for evidence is not to challenge their belief, but to reinforce that these qualities are grounded in real experiences and strengths.)
5. Have your client create a name tag for each adjective (e.g., "Hello, I'm Funny!" "Hello, I'm Kind!" "Hello, I'm Smart!"). Be sure they also create a name tag with their given name so they integrate the idea that these qualities are part of who they are.
6. Allow them to decorate each name tag however they choose.
7. Once the decoration is complete, have them put on the name tags anywhere they want (even silly spots!) and introduce themselves using each name tag. If their caregiver is present, they may also introduce themselves to them.
8. Close by asking how they feel now and what might help them remember to wear those name tags even when they feel tired or discouraged. Remind them that these name tags don't describe every single part of them, but they do present a very awesome and wonderful person: them.

The Story of You

Therapeutic Rationale

We love to use narrative approaches because they are highly versatile, deeply relatable, and meaningful for clients—and they work. Narrative therapy invites kids to reflect on and shape the context of who they are, often for the first time. In this activity, they'll create a third-person narrative of their life story, divided into chapters, to better understand their experiences and explore where they want their story to go next. It can be incredibly helpful for kids, although it is probably not developmentally appropriate for those younger than 13.

Goals

- Reflect on self-concept and examine core beliefs related to the self
- Recapitulate earlier life experiences through an older, wiser lens

Materials

- Writing utensil
- Blank journal or computer writing program

Instructions

1. Ask your client if they have ever wanted to go into "show business." Have they ever wanted to act, write, or direct? If they were writing the story of their life, what would it be about? Would they make it into a book, play, movie, or something else?
2. Explain that you'd like to work together to create the story of their life to help them explore, understand, and work through any difficult experiences they'd had. Share that this is a longer-term project that will take place over one or two sessions.*
3. Explain that this life story will include four basic components:
   a. Birth until two to three years ago
   b. Two to three years ago to about one year ago
   c. About one year ago to the present
   d. Now until the future
4. They should write this narrative in the third person, with an omniscient narrator who knows the main character's (i.e., the client's) thoughts and feelings (e.g., "[*Client's name*] went to school that day. They felt very nervous.").
5. Ask what format they would like to use for their story. It can be a TV show, movie, play, book of short stories or poems, novel, comic book, concept album—be creative!

* We recommend completing most of this activity in session, particularly if the child has a trauma history. Only allow them to work on it at home if you are confident that they will be able to regulate their emotions.

6. Work through the chapters sequentially in a journal or on a computer writing program. While earlier chapters may be revisited later, do not jump ahead before the current chapter is substantially complete.
7. Provide support as the client works through each chapter, helping them process the experience both in real time and during reflection. Ask about any insights, surprises, or emerging themes. Be on the lookout for any moments, outcomes, or details that are particularly unique or unexpected.
8. After each chapter is complete, ask what they learned about themselves, others, or the world. How does this story chapter affect them today? Are there any parts of their story that they might rewrite or reframe from their current perspective?
9. After the first three chapters are complete, have them begin their fourth. What do they want their future to look like? What is important to them? How can you work together to work toward this future?

20 Questions

Therapeutic Rationale

This activity uses a playful and curious format (20 Questions) to help kids explore the distinction between their internal experiences (thoughts, feelings, urges) and their deeper, observing self. By reflecting on different aspects of their experiences, personality, and identity, kids learn that they are not defined by a single feeling, thought, or label. This activity encourages both perspective-taking and self-awareness, which are core components of self-as-context in ACT.

Goals

- Build flexible awareness of self beyond moment-to-moment thoughts or feelings
- Foster curiosity and reflection without judgment
- Strengthen ability to take perspective on inner experiences

Materials

- *20 Questions* handout
- Writing utensil

Instructions

1. Explain that today you'll be playing a version of 20 Questions, but instead of guessing an object, the client will ask themselves questions to better understand who they are. Emphasize that the goal is to notice how many different qualities make up who they are—not just what they're feeling in the moment.
2. Using the *20 Questions* handout, invite the client to answer as many as they can. They don't need to complete all 20 in one sitting.
3. Highlight that some questions relate to feelings, others to actions, and others to memories or values. Reinforce the idea that although all of these qualities are part of the client, *none of them* tell the whole story: "You are way more than just a thought or a feeling. You're the one who notices them all."

20 Questions Handout

1. What is a feeling you've had today?
2. What is something you're good at?
3. What is something that makes you laugh?
4. What do you believe about yourself that might not always be true?
5. What is one thing you love to do?
6. What's a thought you had today that surprised you?
7. What is something you used to think but don't anymore?
8. What is a dream you have for the future?
9. What's a time you felt really proud of yourself?
10. What is something that worries you sometimes?
11. What do your friends or family say they like about you?
12. What's a time you helped someone?
13. What's something you've learned recently?
14. What's a time you felt strong, even when things were hard?
15. What's a thought that comes up a lot but isn't always true?
16. What is something that helps you calm down?
17. What's something about you that no one can see just by looking?
18. What do you value or care about a lot?
19. What's a part of you that you want others to understand better?
20. What's one thing you know is true even when you're sad, mad, or worried?

Elevator Pitch

Therapeutic Rationale

This activity introduces the idea that kids are more than their roles, thoughts, feelings. By asking kids to describe themselves in a short "elevator pitch," they build awareness of a broader, more flexible sense of identity and begin to separate the self from any single experience or label. This activity serves as a practical entry point to explore self-as-context, helping kids begin to notice the observer self—the part of them that has always been there across every stage and feeling.

Goals

- Explore identity beyond roles or surface-level traits
- Promote a flexible self-description and awareness that considers context

Materials

- Blank paper
- Writing utensil
- Stopwatch or timer

Instructions

1. Ask the client to write an elevator pitch about themselves. Explain that an elevator pitch is a short, quick summary they would give if they only had a minute or two to introduce themselves to someone new. What would they say in this pitch?
2. Encourage the client to include multiple aspects of themselves in this elevator pitch rather than just focusing on one or two traits.
3. Have them aim to write 100 words or less, or you can set a timer for two minutes and ask them to write until time is up.
4. When they're done, review the pitch together. What did they notice about themselves? Did anything surprise them? Point out how their pitch reflects more than any single thought, feeling, or role.

Playlist of Me

Therapeutic Rationale

Music is a near-universal human experience, and most people have certain songs that resonate with them and evoke certain feelings. As clinicians, we can use this to help kids explore who they are and what it means to be themselves. We often say to kids, "There are so many labels that can apply to you. You can be tall, funny, kind, smart—you can be anything! Through all of that, the most important label of all is [*client's name*]; let's find out what it means to be [*client's name*]." In this homework activity, kids will create a personalized playlist—"a playlist of me"—that reflects who they are as a person, not just the songs they like.

Goals

- Support clients in reflecting on and expressing their core identity
- Build rapport and validate the client's unique sense of self

Materials

- Computer with speakers

Instructions

1. Ask the client if they have ever listened to or created a playlist of music. What was the playlist for? How did they select the songs on it?
2. Explain that for homework, you would like the client to create another playlist—"a playlist of me"—that reflects who they are as a person, not just their favorite songs. They can include one or two favorite tracks, but no more.
3. In the next session, have them share the playlist with you. For each song, invite them to share why they chose it and what it reflects about who they are. Listen to the song together and thank them for sharing it with you. Validate their music choice and avoid making any judgments (even if a song is "not your style"). If you reject the music, they will feel as though you are rejecting that part of them.
4. Repeat the process for each song. This can continue over several sessions if necessary.
5. Once you have completed the list, ask what the process was like for them. Some questions you could ask include:
   - "What surprised you as you were doing this?"
   - "What was it like for you to share this with me?"
   - "How would you feel about sharing this with anyone else?"
   - "Did you learn or realize anything as a result of doing this? If so, what?"
6. Close the activity by asking what the client would like to take forward and remember from this experience. How can you work together to accomplish that?

Skill Practice and Application

Building LEGO

Therapeutic Rationale

This activity uses LEGO bricks to explore the concept of self-as-context. Each brick represents a part of the child—a feeling, moment, memory, belief, or skill—but no single brick defines who they are. By building a structure from individual pieces, kids can visually and physically experience that while every part of them matters, no single piece *is* the whole structure. This promotes flexible self-awareness and supports defusion from rigid self-labels (e.g., "I'm just an anxious kid").

Goals

- Help clients see themselves as more than any single thought, feeling, or experience
- Promote flexible identity awareness

Materials

- LEGO bricks
- Masking tape and writing utensil (optional)
- Washable marker (optional)

Instructions

1. Introduce the activity: "We're going to build something with LEGO today, but not just for fun. Each piece you choose will represent a part of you. Some pieces might be feelings, some might be memories, and some might be things you're good at. By the end, you'll see that while each piece matters, no one piece is the whole story."
2. Allow the client to begin building, encouraging them to pause and reflect on each brick as they add it. They can label each piece verbally or write directly on the brick using tape or a washable marker. For example:
    - "This piece is when I felt embarrassed last week."
    - "This one is my love of dogs."
    - "This is when I got a bad grade."
    - "This is my creativity."
3. Once the structure is complete, invite the client to name it:
    - "This is me."
    - "This is my story so far."
    - "This is what I'm made of today, but it might look different next week."
4. Let them notice how each part contributed to the final creation.
5. After the activity, offer some reflection prompts. For example:
    - "What was it like to label different parts of yourself with bricks?"

- "Did any piece feel like it didn't belong? Why?"
- "If someone only saw one of your bricks, what might they misunderstand?"
- "What piece are you most proud of including today?"
- "How can you remind yourself that you are always more than just one piece?"

Skill Practice and Application

Invisible Ink Affirmations

Therapeutic Rationale

When kids fuse with unhelpful thoughts (e.g., "I'm bad," "I can't do it," "No one likes me"), it becomes hard for them to see themselves as more than that one thought or feeling. This activity builds self-as-context by helping kids explore and expand their identity beyond the present thought. Just like invisible ink reveals hidden messages when light shines on it, they can "shine a light" on other truths about themselves that might be harder to see but are always there.

Goals

- Step back from thoughts and recognize they are only one part of an experience
- Develop a more flexible and compassionate sense of self
- Notice qualities, values, and truths that can "shine through" even when negative thoughts dominate

Materials

- *Invisible Ink Affirmations* template
- Writing utensil
- White crayon with watercolor paint or UV invisible ink pens (optional)

Instructions

1. Introduce the activity: "Sometimes, when we have a really sticky thought, it can feel like it takes over everything. It's like that thought is all we can see. But there are always other parts of ourselves that are true, even if they are hidden. Today we are going to shine a light on those parts."
2. In the thought bubble at the top of the *Invisible Ink Affirmations* template, have the client write one sticky thought or self-judgment that has been coming up often (e.g., "I'm dumb," "No one wants to be my friend").
3. Ask the client, "What if this thought—which has been so loud that it feels like it's taking up a lot of space—is not the whole picture?"
4. In the flashlight beam on the template, have the client write (or draw) in at least three (but ideally more) "invisible ink" affirmations—truths about themselves that always exist, even when they are hard to see (e.g., "I am learning every day," "I might make mistakes, but I always keep going"). Encourage them to think about compliments they've received from important people, qualities they value about themselves, or times they have acted in a brave, kind, or helpful manner.
5. **Optional:** Use a white crayon or an invisible ink pen to write "invisible" affirmations. As the affirmations are revealed (by painting over the crayon or using the pen's UV light) reinforce, "These things were always there. You just needed to shine your light to see them!"

Invisible Ink Affirmation Template

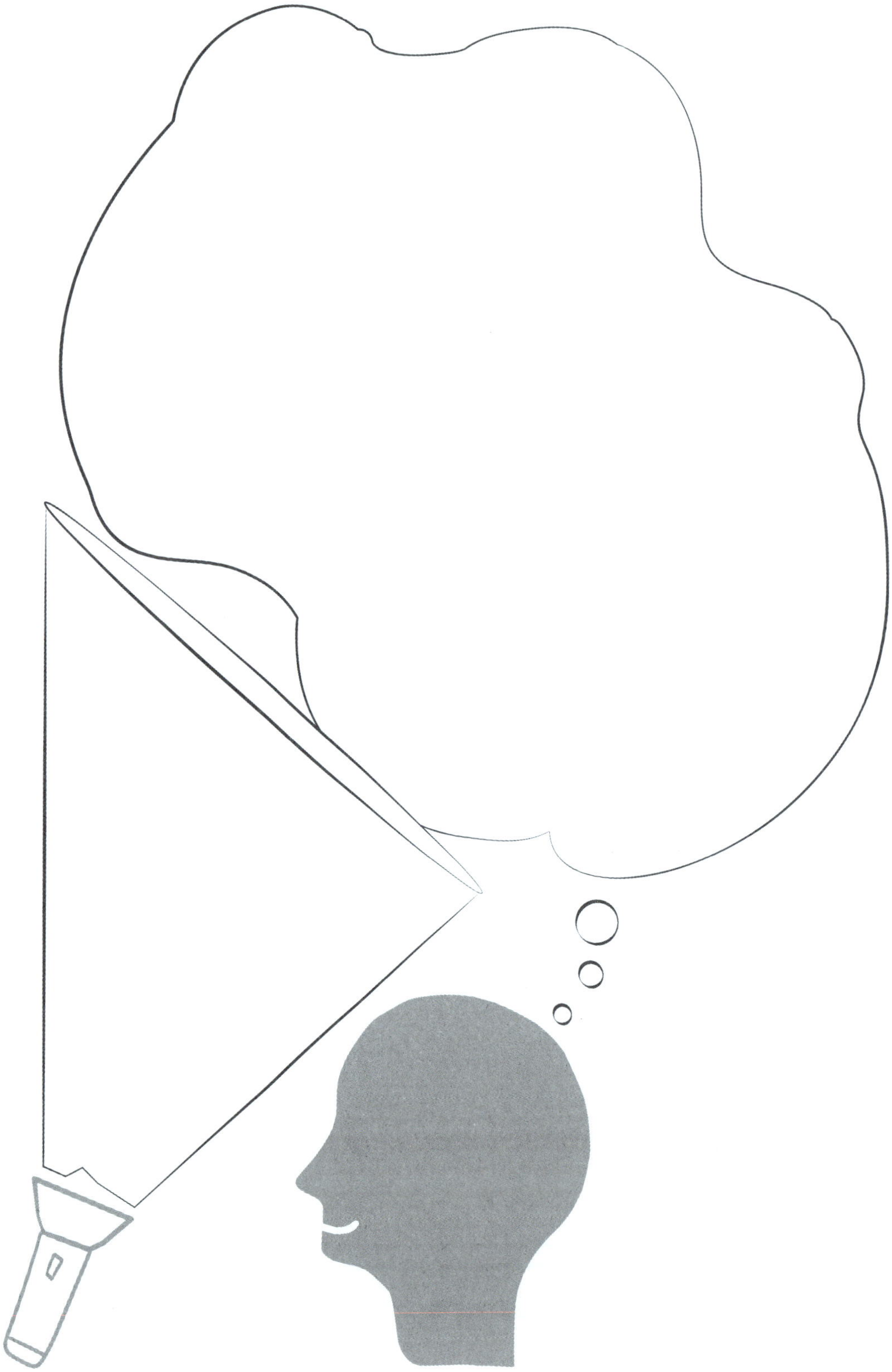

Who I Am, Who I Want to Be: Part 1

Therapeutic Rationale

This activity invites kids to reflect on their evolving sense of self by exploring both who they are now and who they hope to become. From an ACT lens, it supports self-as-context by helping clients gently separate "who I am" from "who I want to be." This creates space for growth, curiosity, and acceptance of all the parts of themselves, including those still in progress. This is a two-part activity, with part 2 found on page 280 in Section 6: Committed Action.

Goals

- Build self-awareness and flexible self-concept
- Separate identity from momentary thoughts, emotions, or struggles
- Foster compassionate self-reflection and values-guided intention

Materials

- *Who I Am, Who I Want to Be* worksheet
- Writing utensil
- Crayons, markers, or colored pencils
- Glue
- Stickers or magazine cutouts

Instructions

1. Introduce the activity: "Sometimes, we get stuck thinking we're only one thing—like *only* shy, *only* silly, or *only* nervous. But in reality, we're always growing and changing. There are things about us that are true right now, and there are also things we're working on becoming. Today we are going to explore both!"
2. On the top half of the *Who I Am, Who I Want to Be* worksheet, have the client write, draw, or collage who they are right now. Consider their qualities, passions, hobbies, and favorite things. If they have a hard time getting started, you may offer a few prompts:
   - "I am someone who . . ."
   - "Right now I care a lot about . . ."
   - "People describe me as . . ."
   - "I would describe myself as . . ."
3. On the bottom half, have them write, draw, or collage who they *want* to be someday. What kind of friend, sibling, student, or person do they want to become? Encourage aspirational thinking. This is not about perfection, but direction. Prompts may include:
   - "I want to be someone who . . ."
   - "In the future, I hope I can . . ."
   - "Even when things are hard, I want to keep being . . ."
   - "If I could describe my best self, that person would be . . ."

Who I Am, Who I Want to Be Worksheet

In the spaces below, represent who you are now and who you want to be.

Who I Am

Who I Want to Be

Skill Practice and Application

Where Do You Sit in the Theater?

Therapeutic Rationale

Learned helplessness can make kids feel stuck, even when they have all of the tools to reach their goals. It is amazing how often "I can't" actually means "I won't." This activity uses the theater as a metaphor to help kids explore the roles they play (or choose not to play) in their own lives. By reflecting on whether they are passive observers, active performers, or directors of their own story, kids can gain insight into their sense of agency and seek opportunities for change.

Goals

- Reflect on personal agency
- Recognize the roles clients play in their own lives
- Instill a sense of autonomy and self-efficacy

Materials

- *Theater* template
- Writing utensil
- Crayons, markers, or colored pencils

Instructions

1. Begin by sharing with William Shakespeare's quote: "All the world's a stage." Ask the client what that means to them and take some time to explore roles that your client plays in their life. Do they watch people on stage as a passive observer? Are they one of the performers on stage? Are they the director? Does their role change depending on the situation?
2. Introduce the *Theater* template and invite them to write or draw times in their life where they have played the following roles:
   a. **A performer:** When they take action (e.g., practice a sport)
   b. **An audience member:** When they are a passive observer (e.g., not speaking up in class)
   c. **A director:** When they guide events behind the scenes (e.g., helping a friend handle a tricky situation with a peer)
3. How do they feel about their placement in the theater?
   a. Are they content being on the stage, in the audience, or in the background? Why or why not?
   b. What steps can they take collaboratively with you to move forward with those changes?
4. This is a helpful metaphor and conversation to come back to—use your best judgment!

Theater Template

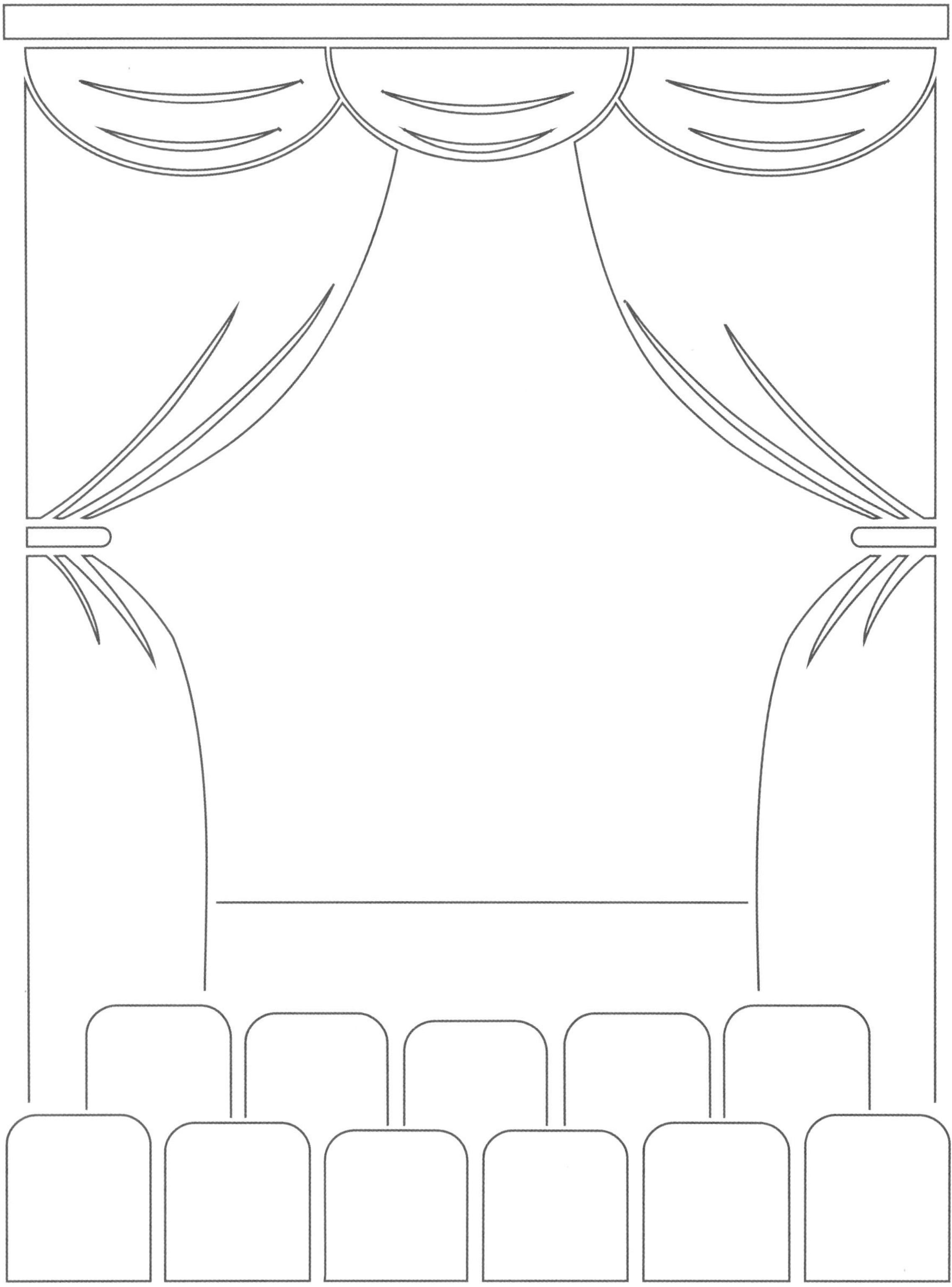

I'm Not That . . . Part 1

Therapeutic Rationale

This activity helps kids build distance from harsh, self-critical thoughts, like "I'm not smart," "No one likes me," or "I'll never be good at this." While it's common for kids to have thoughts like this from time to time, self-as-context teaches that we are not defined by the content of our thoughts, but that we are the ones noticing those thoughts. By borrowing from a classic literature activity—where students explore who the characters *are*—this activity encourages kids to reflect on who they truly are, as opposed to what their thoughts tell them.

Goals

- Build a flexible and compassionate self-narrative
- Highlight overlooked strengths and traits
- Observe thoughts instead of being defined by them

Materials

- *Traits Word Bank* handout
- Writing utensil

Instructions

1. Introduce the activity: "Sometimes, we have an inner voice that tells us things like 'I'm dumb' or 'I'm not good enough.' But these are just thoughts—they don't define who we really are. If we're *not* those things, then who are we? Today we're going to explore that together."
2. Provide your client with the *Traits Word Bank* handout, which includes many examples of traits that someone, anyone, might hold. Have them go through the list and circle traits that best describe them. You can also create your own word bank or build off the one provided as a starting point.
3. Conclude the activity by reflecting together. Which traits felt most accurate or surprising to see? Are there qualities they hadn't noticed about themselves before? What does it feel like to notice these traits while remembering that they are not defined by self-critical thoughts?
4. **Optional:** Invite the client's caregiver to complete the activity at the same time by circling the traits they feel describe the child. Once they have both finished, compare the similarities and differences. This allows the client to see how others see and describe them.

Traits Word Bank Handout

Curious

Determined

Brave

Friendly

Loyal

Caring

Calm

Goofy

Thoughtful

Imaginative

Sensitive

Adventurous

Kind

Creative

Helpful

Smart

Funny

Athletic

Honest

Hardworking

Silly

Skill Practice and Application

I'm Not That . . . Part 2

Therapeutic Rationale

This follow-up activity invites children to externalize and visualize the many descriptive parts of themselves within a silhouette. Kids will examine the traits, thoughts, and self-descriptions they identified in part 1 of this activity and then "size" them based on how prominent each one feels in their current self-view. This visual self-map supports self-as-context by showing that we are not any single trait or thought, but a collection of many evolving parts. Traits may grow or shrink over time, so none of them define us completely.

Goals

- Reinforce flexible, compassionate identity-building
- Develop self-awareness of how personal characteristics shift over time

Materials

- *Traits Word Bank* handout (completed)
- *Silhouette* template
- Writing utensil
- Crayons, markers, or colored pencils
- Craft items (e.g., stickers, glitter, glue)

Instructions

1. Begin by looking back at the *Traits Word Bank* handout (see page 160). Have the client reflect on which traits feel like major parts of their identity today, which traits are smaller but still present, and whether there are any they'd like to remove or add.
2. Guide the client to use the *Silhouette* template to show all the different parts of themselves. Have them write or draw each trait inside the body, sizing each according to how big or small it feels to their self-view today.
3. Encourage them to decorate or highlight the words in ways that reflect what they mean to them. There is no right or wrong way to do this, as it is a reflection of who the client is right now. All of these pieces within them can change and grow over time.
4. Ask the client to consider what happens when a negative or mean thought tries to take up too much space. Remind them that just like other traits, these thoughts can change over time—they may feel bigger or smaller on different days. Emphasize that they can acknowledge these thoughts without getting stuck in them, knowing that the thoughts won't always stay the same size.

Silhouette Template

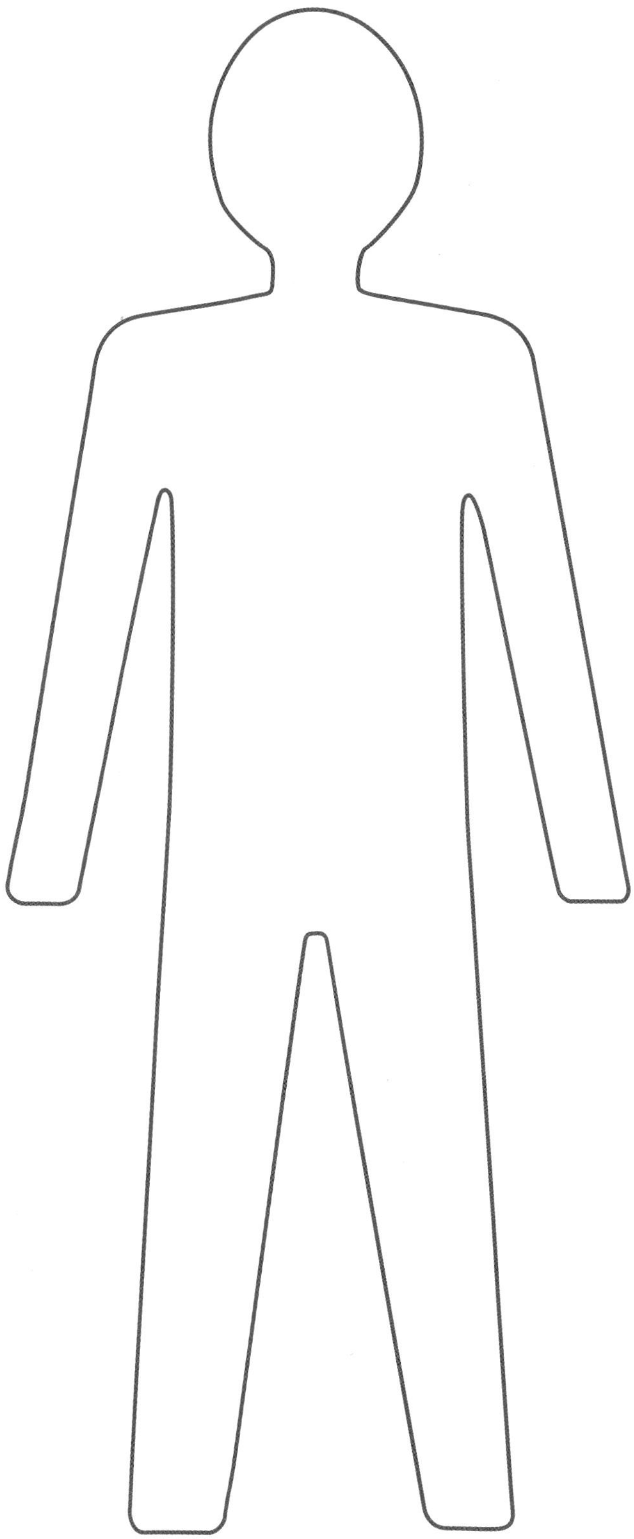

What Fills My Well?

Therapeutic Rationale

It's often said that you cannot pour from an empty cup. To take the metaphor one step further, where do we get the water to refill our cup? From a well, of course—our well of internal and external resources, skills, and coping strategies that we call on when needed. However, some of those resources are more available at certain times than others. For example, it is snowing as we write this, and while we both love taking our dogs to the park on a sunny day, the current weather makes that more difficult. This activity is designed to help kids conceptualize, recall, and actively use the resources, skills, and coping strategies at their disposal.

Goals

- Recall relevant resources, skills, and coping strategies
- Reinforce the importance of self-care and refilling the client's "cup"

Materials

- *Self-Care Well* template
- Writing utensil

Instructions

1. Ask your client if they have ever heard the phrase "You can't pour from an empty cup," and explore what it means: You need to take care of yourself before you can take care of others.
2. Ask your client to reflect on how well they currently refill their own cup. What helps them recharge, rest, and recuperate?
3. Together, write down all of the ways your client can refill their cup in the water reservoir section of the *Self-Care Well* template. Discuss when and how it might be appropriate to use different resources or strategies.
4. Invite the client to consider the size of their water reservoir. Is it big enough? Do they need to fill it with more skills, strategies, or resources? Work with them to develop additional resources if needed.
5. Explore how your client feels about prioritizing self-care. Do they ever feel guilt or shame about it? If so, why? Where did they learn that it is "wrong" to fill their own cup first?
6. Conclude by collaborating on a self-care plan for the coming week, writing it down in the designated section of the template. Assign this plan for homework.

Self-Care Well Template

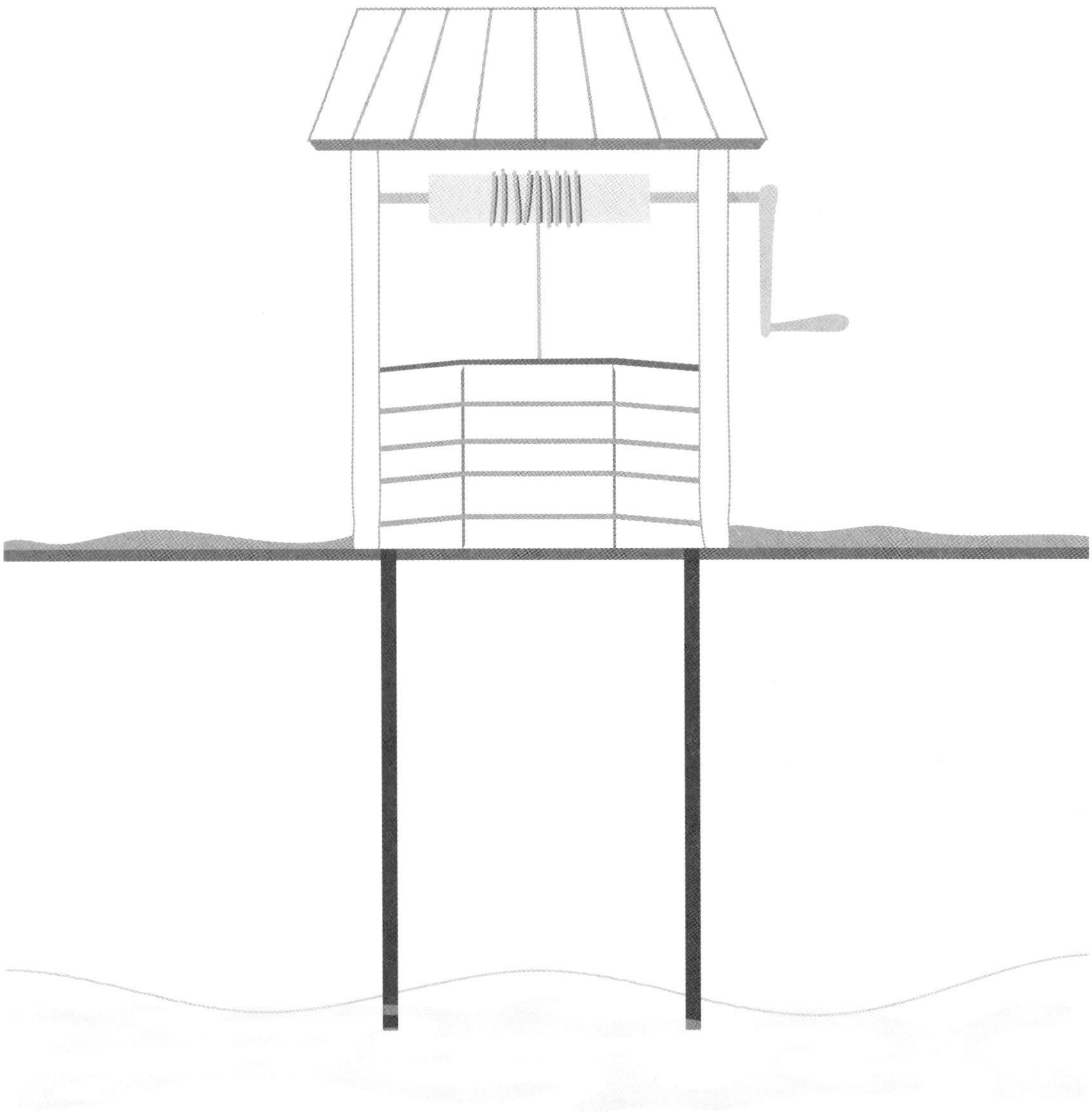

My Self-Care Action Plan

____

____

____

____

____

Skill Practice and Application

What Fuels My Fire?

Therapeutic Rationale

Many kids come into our offices hoping that therapy will make life easy. Unfortunately, that is not the case. Therapy does not prevent the hard stuff from being hard. What therapy *can* do is help kids recognize and strengthen their internal resources so they can draw upon them when the going gets tough. This activity uses the metaphor of a flame to represent those internal resources and strengths. When kids face stress, pressure, or situations that pull them away from a values-driven life, it's easier stay grounded when their inner flame is well-fueled. In this activity, kids will identify what fuels the fire of that flame and keeps it burning.

Goals

- Increase awareness of internal sources of strength and resilience
- Support clients in recognizing their own power and autonomy

Materials

- *Fire* template
- Writing utensil
- Crayons, markers, or colored pencils
- Scissors
- Sandwich baggie

Instructions

1. Ask your client to recall a time when they got through something difficult. What was that like for them? What allowed them to persevere?
2. Use this as a starting point to introduce the idea of resiliency as the ability to persevere and make it through, even when things are challenging. Compare resiliency to a flame inside us that provides warmth, energy, and strength. Explain that this flame can be fueled by many things, such as values, beliefs, hopes, memories, love, and coping skills.
3. Ask your client how brightly their resiliency flame burns. What keeps it burning?
4. On the logs on the *Fire* template, have your client write down different values, beliefs, hopes, memories, or other sources of strength. Encourage them to choose smaller or larger pieces depending on how much strength each source provides.
5. Have the client color in the flame and logs, then cut out the logs.
6. Apply the flame metaphor to recent challenges the client is experiencing. Which "logs" do they need to add to their fire to help keep it burning? How can they find more logs (i.e., sources of fuel) to keep the fire going? Discuss when smaller logs may be enough and when larger logs are necessary.
7. Have the client put their logs (and some blank ones) in a baggie to take home as a reminder to them of their own strength and resiliency they can draw on when things feel hard.

Fire Template

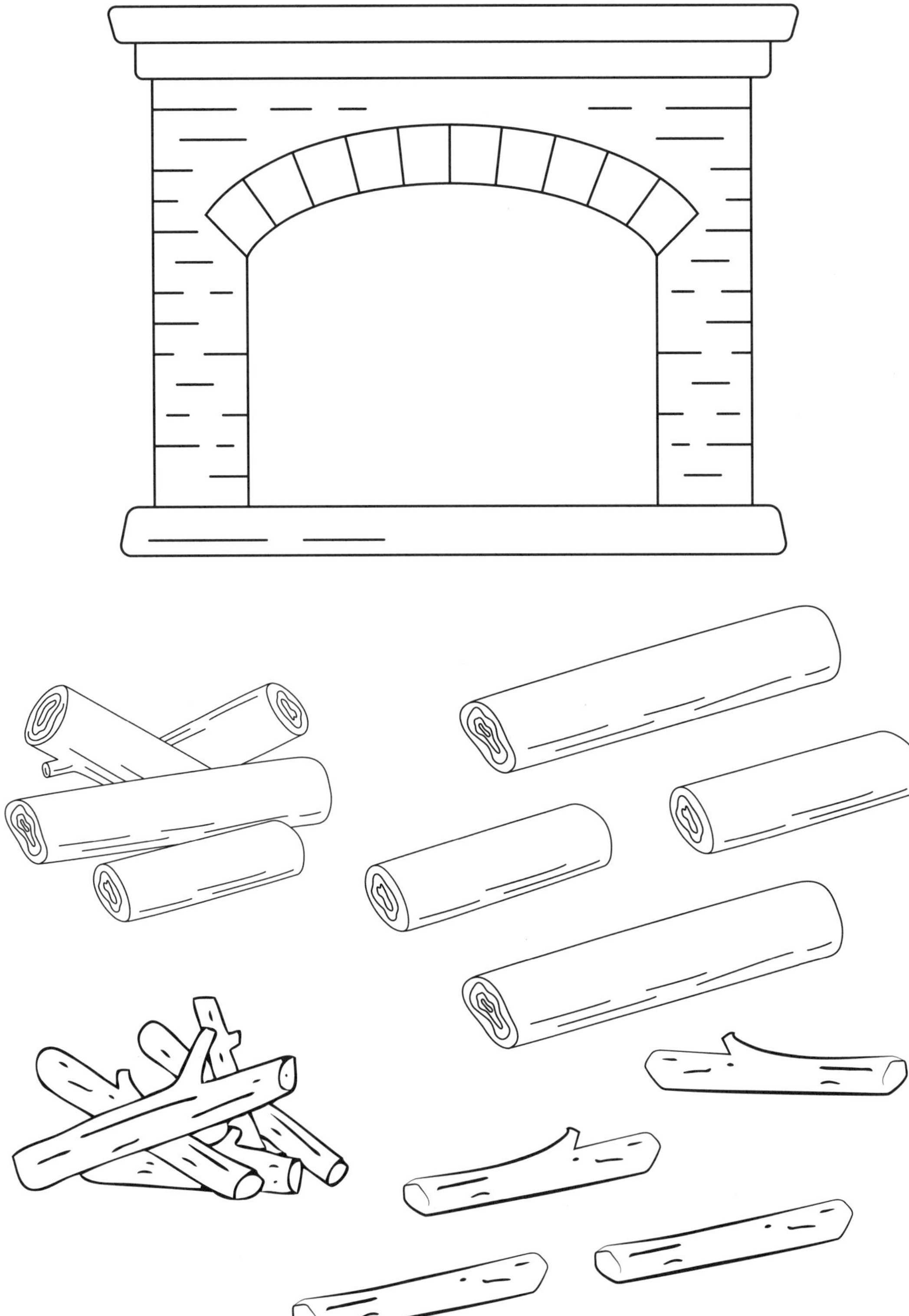

Empty Chair

Therapeutic Rationale

One of the strengths of ACT is its compatibility with other theoretical models. In many ways, it's almost a metamodel of psychological flexibility! We are able to incorporate elements of other modalities and psychological traditions that fit particular cases or clients, which is incredibly helpful. In this activity, we borrow the empty chair technique from Gestalt therapy and give it our own ACT twist.

Goals

- Externalize thoughts as a means to gain insight into the true nature of distress
- Provide a safe, nonreactive way to express emotions

Materials

- An empty chair or couch

Instructions

1. When your client is upset, work with them to identify who or what they are upset at. This can be a person, a situation, an emotion, or even an abstract concept (e.g., a parent's illness, life itself).
2. Ask the client to visualize that person or thing sitting in the chair in front of them. Invite the client to describe what that person or thing looks like and what their presence feels like.*
3. Encourage your client to say whatever they need to say to the chair. This may take some encouragement. Reassure them the chair cannot react to what they say and that as soon as the session ends, whatever they said will be forgotten—allowing your client to speak freely. Let them know that there's no need to filter themselves or hold back. They can let it all out!
4. Once your client has said everything they need to say, help them ground themselves back in the present moment (e.g., noticing their breath, feeling their feet on the floor).
5. What was this experience like for them? What surprised them? What did they discover about their thoughts or feelings? Are they actually upset with who or what they initially thought? If not, who or what are they actually upset with? How do they want this experience to inform their actions moving forward?
6. The entire experience is a method to gain insight into the self, so this ending reflection and processing is the most critical element. It is vital that you give them time!

---

* If you are performing this intervention virtually, we recommend turning your camera off and changing your name on the screen to match the name of the identified person or thing. That way, your client will see a black box with the name in it. We've found this to be very effective.

Growing Resilience

Therapeutic Rationale

Self-as-context helps kids notice that they are not just their thoughts, feelings, or labels—they are the container that holds them all. This multi-session activity uses the metaphor of a growing plant to illustrate that people, like plants, are always changing. Just as a bean seed grows into a sprout and eventually a full plant, kids can begin to see themselves as something bigger than any single moment, struggle, or label.

Goals

- Normalize and accept ongoing growth and change
- Explore identity as an evolving process rather than a fixed story
- Emphasize that we are more than our thoughts or feelings

Materials

- Dry bean seeds
- Small cup or pot with soil
- Water and access to sunlight or a window
- Craft supplies (e.g., paint, markers, stickers, glue, glitter) to decorate the pot (optional)

Instructions

1. Introduce the concept of growth by explaining that people, like plants, grow and change over time. In this way, we are not just our thoughts or feelings. We are so much more than that, and we are continually growing and moving toward our goals.
2. Have the client plant the bean seed in soil using a small pot or cup. Invite them to decorate the pot in a way that represents themselves, such as their interests, strengths, or personality.
3. Across multiple sessions, observe and reflect on the plant together:
    a. "What does the seed or plant look like now? Has anything changed since last time?"
    b. "Even if we can't see it, what is happening under the soil?"
    c. "How is this similar to people and their thoughts or feelings?"
4. Between sessions, be sure to water the plant regularly and, if helpful, take photos of the changes to share with the client. Reinforce that growing a plant, like moving toward our goals, takes time, care, and effort.
5. As the seed sprouts, reflect on how the seed is still part of the plant, but it is no longer *just* a seed. Normalize that where it started is not "wrong"; it was simply one stage of growth.
6. Continue using the growing plant as a metaphor for the client's experience:
    a. "You are not just one version of yourself. Like the seed becoming a sprout, you're always growing."
    b. "Just because you're feeling ____ today doesn't mean that's all you are."

Ripples in the Water: Part 1

Therapeutic Rationale

This metaphor-based activity uses the visual of ripples in water to help kids reflect on the people, influences, and experiences that shape who they are. The key is that we are not defined by any single ripple. Just as ripples expand, fade, and overlap, our relationships and inner experiences shift and evolve. By helping kids identify who and what is in their circle—and noticing which ripples feel closer to the center or farther away—they begin to notice their sense of self in relation to others, which fosters perspective-taking and self-as-context. This is a two-part activity, with part 2 found on page 236 in Section 5: Values.

Goals

- Promote perspective-taking and flexible identity
- Externalize social, emotional, and relational influences

Materials

- *Ripple* template
- Writing utensil
- Bucket with water and a small stone or object (optional)

Instructions

1. Introduce the metaphor by explaining that when a pebble is thrown into a pond, it creates ripples that move outward in circles. Sometimes, new things land in the water and make new ripples too. Connect this to the client's experience by explaining that when certain things happen in life (unexpectedly or otherwise)—like people, events, or unkind thoughts—the ripple they create shows what has the biggest impact on us and what matters most.
2. Optionally, you can demonstrate this by throwing a small stone into a bucket of water and highlighting how the ripples move outward.
3. Explain that this activity is about noticing who and what creates ripples in their life, and how close or far away those ripples feel right now.
4. On the *Ripple* template, ask the client to write their name in the center circle where it says "Me." Then have them add people, places, experiences, thoughts, emotions, or memories to the surrounding rings based on how close, important, or impactful they feel.
5. As the client fills out the template, offer some discussion prompts. For example:
    - "Who or what makes big waves in your life right now?"
    - "Who do you feel closest to?"

- "Are there any ripples that feel hard or heavy? Any that feel light?"
- "Have any ripples changed size or moved closer or farther away over time?"

6. Revisit this activity periodically to notice what has changed, including the placement of the ripples.

Ripple Template

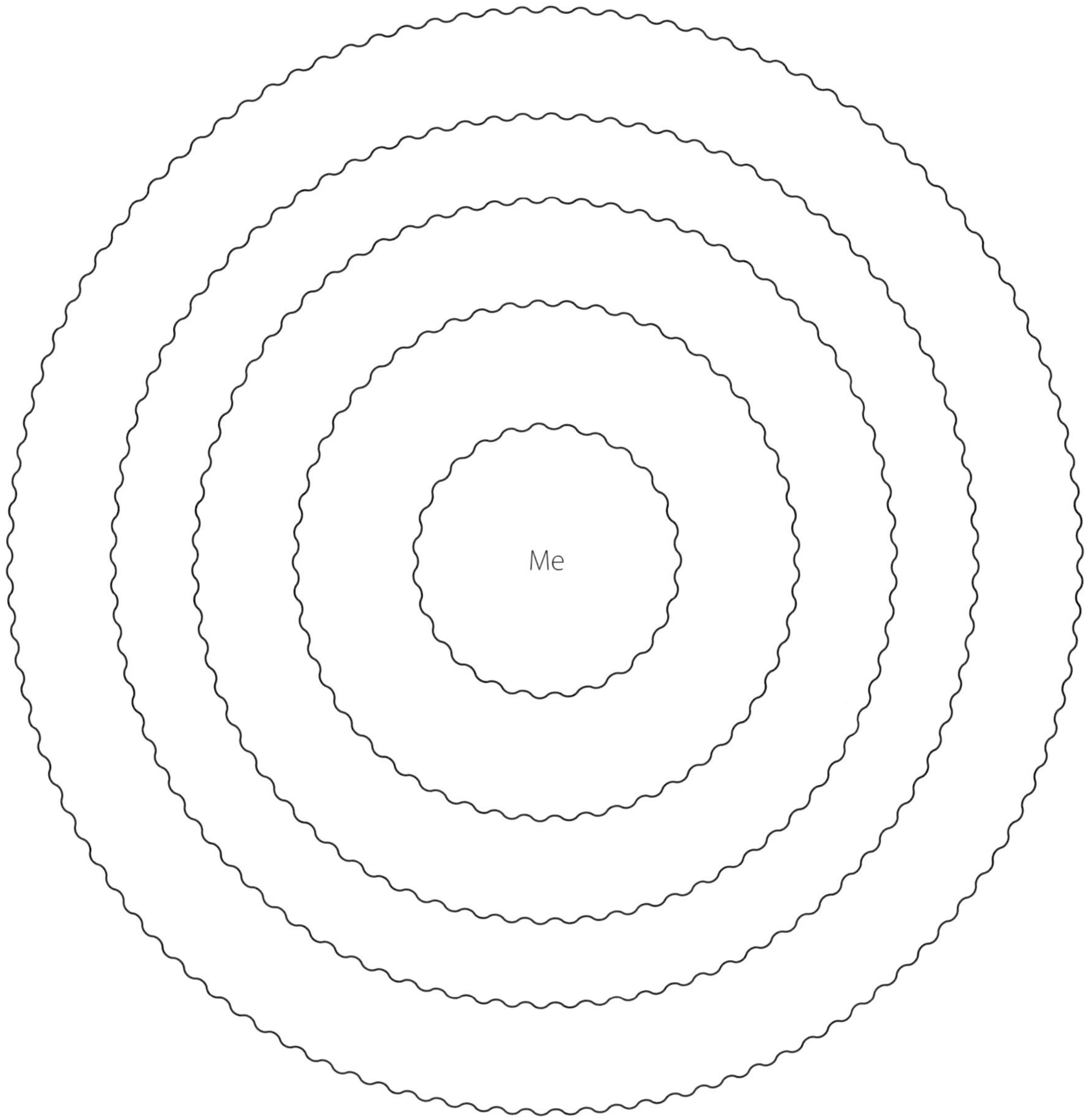

Core Memories

Therapeutic Rationale

In the film *Inside Out*, the main character, Riley, has core memories that shape her as a person. This activity invites kids to identify their own core memories and reflect on how each experience has shaped them. By examining both the helpful and unhelpful lessons they've learned from these memories, they can gain perspective on how their past has shaped them, and what's more, how they want these experiences to shape them moving forward. This activity draws from narrative therapy by encouraging kids to identify unique or noteworthy outcomes of their narrative. Note that this exercise may not be appropriate for clients who have experienced significant unprocessed trauma.

Goals

- Promote reflection and insight
- Facilitate a stronger sense of self and identity
- View core memories (both helpful and unhelpful) as components of the whole

Materials

- Blank paper
- Writing utensil

Instructions

1. Ask your client if they have seen the film *Inside Out*. If not, suggest watching it with their caregivers as homework.
2. Invite them to recall what it was like inside Riley's head: the emotions, thoughts, and core memories that make her who she is. What did they notice about these different elements? How did they all interact? Were they always helpful to Riley, or did they sometimes get into trouble while trying to protect her?
3. Explain that today you want to focus on the client's core memories—the experiences that have fundamentally shaped who they are.
4. Work together to create a list of five to seven of the client's core memories. Emphasize that these are not necessarily "good" or "bad" memories—they're just the experiences that have had the most significant impact on their life.
5. For each memory, ask the client to describe what happened, what they felt and thought at the time, and how they reacted. Discuss the lessons each memory may have taught them about themselves, others, and the world. Were these lessons helpful or unhelpful? Could a different perspective provide a more helpful takeaway? For example, if a client was bullied and concluded "All people are mean," a more adaptive lesson might be "Some people are mean, but I can protect myself and find supportive relationships."

6. Make sure to approach sensitive memories with care. If any experience seems especially powerful or distressing, pause the activity to help the client regulate their emotions.
7. As a closing reflection, ask your client to consider how these core memories have collectively shaped their sense of self. What lessons have they learned about themselves when it comes to their kindness, empathy, and resilience?

Casting Your Life

Therapeutic Rationale

Who hasn't, at some point, considered which actor might play them in a movie about their life? Matt is convinced (despite all evidence to the contrary) that only a young Clark Gable could portray him, while Emily would best be portrayed by June Squibb. Just as actors take on different roles, we also play a variety of roles in our lives and in the lives of others. This activity helps kids reflect on the roles they play, determine what roles are most important to them, and consider what roles they want to play moving forward.

Goals

- Gain insight into personal roles and how they shape experiences
- Encourage honest self-reflection using familiar pop-culture references

Materials

- Blank paper
- Writing utensil

Instructions

1. Invite your client to play a game of pretend. You want to figure out who would be the best person to portray them in a movie or TV show about their life.
2. Have your client write out the roles that will need to be cast beyond themselves: parents, siblings, friends, relatives, caregivers—anyone who is important to them.
3. Once they have determined the roles, start brainstorming! Who should play each role and why? What about that person would best represent the client or their loved ones? What do they see in that actor that reflects the quality of the person they are portraying? Have them write down their cast list on a piece of paper.
4. For younger kiddos (or clients who don't know a lot of actor names), you can allow the use of fictional characters. You can also have the client list multiple actors or characters for each role and explain why each fits (e.g., "This person seems kind like me").
5. Once they have created their cast list, guide them through the following prompts:
    a. "What roles do you currently play in your life (e.g., friend, student, sibling)?"
    b. "What roles would you like to play in your life?"
    c. "What is keeping you from playing those desired roles? What obstacles might you need to navigate?"
    d. "What actions can you take so you can play those roles consistently?"
6. When they're done, reflect with your client. What was it like for them to go through this exercise? Are they satisfied with their selections? Which parts were easy or challenging?

Salad Bowl

Therapeutic Rationale

This activity helps kids externalize and reflect on the many different aspects of their identity using the metaphor of a salad. Just like a salad is made up of different ingredients, people are made up of various traits, experiences, emotions, and values. In this activity, kids will learn that they are not defined by any one "ingredient" and that they have agency in noticing, accepting, or even adjusting what elements make up their unique mix.

Goals

- Promote self-awareness and the formation of a flexible identity
- Encourage reflection on internal and external traits, thoughts, and experiences

Materials

- *Salad* template
- Writing utensil
- Crayons, markers, or colored pencils

Instructions

1. Begin by asking the client what they believe a salad is. Most will likely mention lettuce, vegetables, and dressing.
2. Then, expand the conversation: What if it were a fruit salad? Or maybe even a candy salad? Who decides what qualifies a salad? Explain that if a salad is simply a bowl of ingredients eaten together, then almost anything can be a salad.
3. Connect this to the client's identity by explaining, "If you really think about it, our brains (and who we are) are kind of like a salad. We're a mix of many different things that come together to make us who we are. We are not just one ingredient—we're the whole salad."
4. Using the *Salad* template, have the client write or draw the traits, interests, emotions, experiences, and values that feel like a part of them right now inside the bowl. Around the outside of the bowl, they can draw additional "ingredients" that others might have snuck into their salad (like unkind thoughts or unwanted comments from others).
5. Invite the client to reflect on what they want to keep in their salad and what they want to leave out. Encourage them to erase or draw a line through the items they don't want to include moving forward. Remind them that, like a real salad, they can customize the ingredients and leave out the ones that don't serve them.

Salad Template

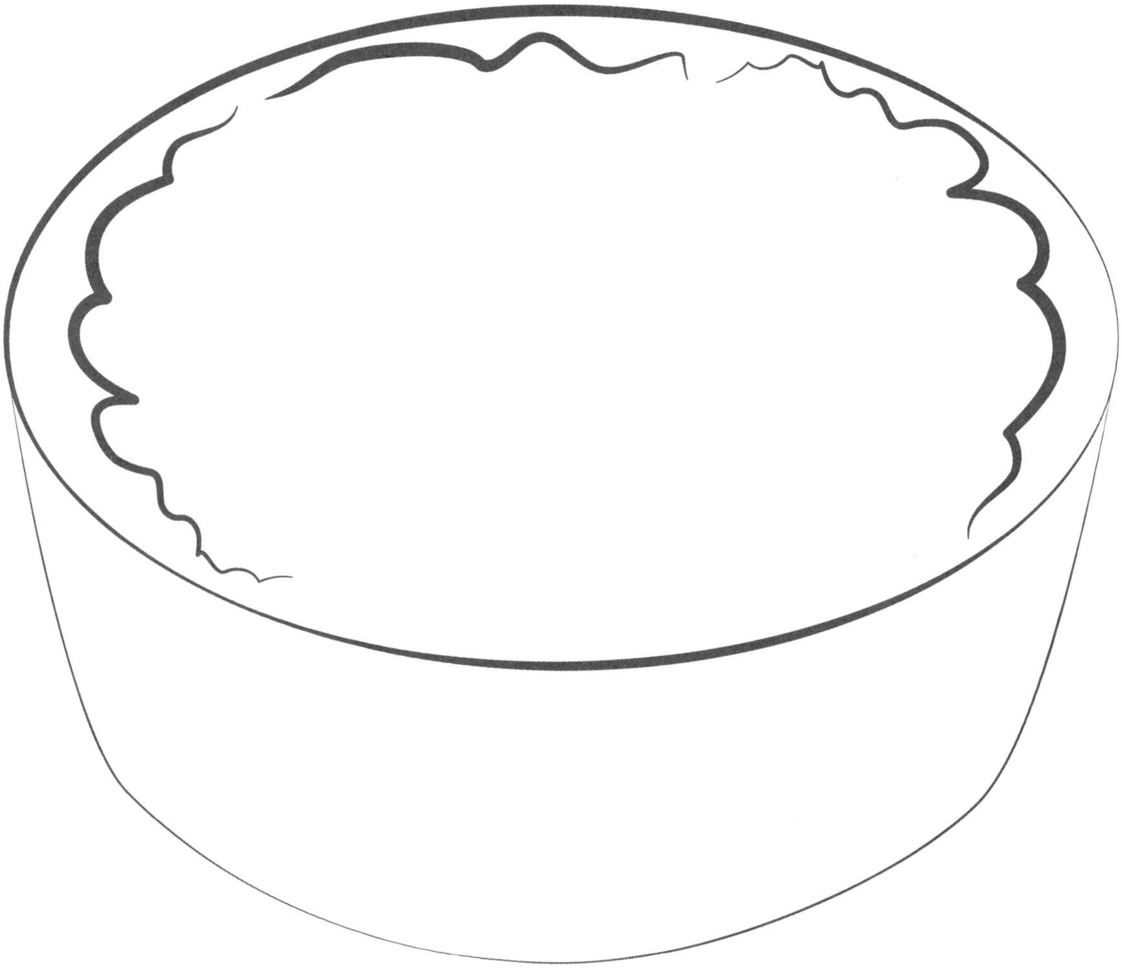

Being Kind to Your Friend: You

Therapeutic Rationale

This activity draws on mindful self-compassion to help kids recognize and observe harsh self-talk. By flipping the script and imagining how they would treat a close friend in the same situation, they learn to notice their internal dialogue and shift toward kinder, more supportive self-talk. This activity also encourages development of the observer self—the part of us that notices thoughts without being defined by them.

Goals

- Increase mindful awareness of negative self-talk
- Foster a compassionate sense of self
- Promote the development of the observer self

Materials

- *Dear Friend* template
- Writing utensil

Instructions

1. Introduce the activity: "Today you are going to write a letter to yourself—but from the perspective of a close friend. In the letter, you'll respond to a situation where you've been feeling self-critical or upset."
2. Guide the client to choose the topic of the letter. Perhaps it's a recent mistake they made, a time they felt disappointed, a situation that made them feel sad, or a self-critical thought that they often struggle with.
3. Encourage them to write the letter as if they *are* that close friend: "What would your best friend say to you in this situation? How would they say it? What would they want you to know?"
4. Make sure the letter addresses the specific situation or feeling (e.g., "I know you felt disappointed when you missed the winning shot for your soccer team, but here's what I want you to know. . .").
5. When they're done, have them read it aloud. Reflect on how it feels to hear those kind words. How does it impact their self-critical thoughts?

Dear Friend Template

Dear Friend,

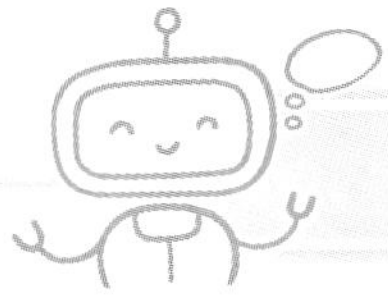

Who, What, Where, When, Why, and How?

Therapeutic Rationale

This activity invites kids to mindfully observe their thoughts through structured reflection. By using the familiar "who, what, where, when, why, and how" framework, kids learn to slow down, notice the details of their thoughts, and gain distance from sticky or overwhelming thoughts. This helps them see themselves as the observer of their thoughts rather than being defined by them.

Goals

- Develop language for self-reflection and thought exploration
- Step back from thoughts and build self-as-context
- Foster emotional flexibility and nonjudgmental noticing

Materials

- *Who, What, Where, When, Why, and How* worksheet
- Writing utensil

Instructions

1. Introduce the idea of guided self-reflection: "Sometimes, our thoughts might seem like they are shouting at us, or like they're sticky glue that we can't get off our hands. While that might be true, we don't have to believe everything we think—and perhaps more importantly, we are not our thoughts. Today we're going to practice slowing down, getting curious, and simply observing the different parts of a thought."
2. Have the client pick a thought to explore. It may be helpful to start with a silly or lighter thought (e.g., "I want grilled cheese for lunch") to help the client feel more comfortable with the concept. Later, they can move on to bigger, stickier thoughts.
3. Walk the client through the *Who, What, Where, When, Why, and How* worksheet, explaining each question:
   a. Who is this thought about? (Is it about you, someone else, or something else?)
   b. What is the thought actually saying? (State it in simple, nonjudgmental language.)
   c. Where in your mind or body do you notice this thought? (e.g., head, stomach, heart)
   d. When do you notice this thought the most? (e.g., at school, at home, before bed)
   e. Why might this thought be showing up? (What are possible reasons or triggers?)
   f. How can you notice this thought without letting it take over? (e.g., step back, observe it, let it pass)
4. After completing the worksheet, ask how it felt to notice the thought in this way. How did it feel to look at the thought as something they can observe rather than something that controls them?

Who, What, Where, When, Why, and How Worksheet

Use the following questions to practice exploring a single thought.

Who is the thought about?

___

What is this thought saying?

___

Where is this thought showing up or coming from?

___

When do you notice this thought the most?

___

Why might you be having this thought?

___

How can you notice this thought without letting it take over?

___

Mindfulness

Self-Talk Switch

Therapeutic Rationale

This activity helps kids observe and reflect on their self-talk by comparing it to how they would speak to a close friend—or how a close friend might respond to them. Often, negative self-talk goes unchecked until it's seen from another point of view. This activity also supports the development of self-as-context by teaching kids to notice their thoughts without fusing to them and to practice kinder, more flexible responses.

Goals

- Foster compassionate self-reflection
- Observe internal dialogue without fusing to it

Materials

- *Self-Talk Switch* worksheet
- Writing utensil

Instructions

1. Explain that sometimes we say things to ourselves that we would never say to our best friend. Let the client know that this activity is about noticing that self-talk and seeing it through the perspective of a close friend.
2. Introduce the *Self-Talk Switch* worksheet, which has three columns:
   a. **What I say to myself:** A thought the client says to themselves
   b. **What I would say to my friend:** What they would tell their friend if they were in that situation
   c. **What my friend might say to me:** What their friend might actually say in response to the client's self-talk
3. Encourage the client to fill out at least three rows with different thoughts. Use the example in the first row to model how to complete the remaining columns.
4. If the client struggles to come up with what a close friend might say, prompt them with questions like "What would you hope to hear from a friend?" or "What might your caregivers say?"
5. After completing the worksheet, ask which responses felt the most supportive or helpful. How does it feel to see their thoughts from another perspective?

Self-Talk Switch Worksheet

Notice a thought you say to yourself, then write down what you would say to a friend in that situation and what a friend might say to you.

What I Say to Myself	What I Would Say to My Friend	What My Friend Might Say to Me
I'm so bad at math.	You're just learning. It's okay not to be perfect.	You've been trying your best and that's what matters most.

Glitter Jar

Therapeutic Rationale

Who doesn't love shiny things? Emily knows that a great way to distract Matt is to find a sparkly object and wave it around. In this activity, kids will have an opportunity to practice mindfulness by observing swirling glitter in water, which represents their thoughts and feelings. Watching the glitter settle helps kids see that their thoughts and feelings can move and change—and they can observe those experiences without being swept away.

Goals

- Introduce mindfulness and self-as-context in a playful, hands-on way
- Observe thoughts and feelings without getting overwhelmed by them

Materials

- Small sealable plastic jar
- Water
- Food dye
- Glitter
- Waterproof tape

Instructions

1. Set up the materials and let your client choose what they want to include in their jar. Remind them that with both food dye and glitter, less is more.
2. Add the materials to their container, then help them secure the lid and tape it closed. Remind them that even though it is sealed, the jar is still fragile.
3. Encourage your client to shake the jar and explore the movement of the glitter.
4. Ask them to describe what they notice. They might respond with "the color" or "the glitter," but prompt them to look deeper: What *else* do they notice, beyond the obvious?
5. Explain that just like the glitter, thoughts and feelings can swirl around inside us, but we are not those thoughts or feelings. We are like the jar—noticing what is happening inside without being swept away by it.
6. Guide the client to practice this kind of noticing in your office. Encourage them to observe their own thoughts, feelings, and bodily sensations as they watch the jar, noticing without trying to control or change them.
7. Encourage them to continue practicing at home with the glitter jar to notice their thoughts, feelings, and body sensations.

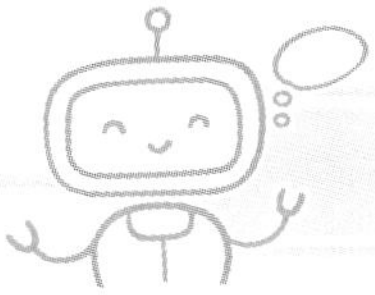

I Spy

Therapeutic Rationale

Many adults have experienced the spark of panic that comes when their child says, "I'm bored!" Our kiddos usually hate to be bored and often struggle when they do not have a stimulating activity or distraction. I Spy, which is a game that most of us have played on long car trips, is often our first, albeit unintentional, introduction to mindfulness. We can use that to our advantage! This adapted version of I Spy transforms the familiar childhood game into an opportunity to practice self-as-context by allowing kids to observe their internal experiences from a place of curiosity, not judgment. Rather than identifying *with* their boredom or frustration, they begin to observe these experiences as passing aspects and small pieces of themselves. In this way, they learn that they are more than one thought, feeling, or moment—they are the noticer of all of it!

Goals

- Practice mindfulness and present-moment awareness
- Develop self-regulation skills when experiencing boredom

Materials

- None

Instructions

1. Explain that traditionally, I Spy is a competitive game. One person says, "I spy with my little eye . . . something that is __________," and the other person guesses the object. However, for this activity, the client will play individually, with a focus on *noticing* rather than guessing.
2. Have your client quietly identify an object in your office or (ideally) outside through the window. Have them quietly say to themselves, "I spy with my little eye . . . something that is ________," describing a quality of the object (e.g., color, shape, size, texture).
3. Next, have the client try to find as many other objects as they can that share that quality. For example, if the object they choose is a plant, they might notice all the plants they can see. If they choose a blue object, they can count all the blue objects.
4. After a few rounds, introduce the idea of noticing their internal experiences. For example, "I spy with my little eye . . . a part of me that feels tense." What other parts of them feel tense? Can they practice noticing those parts? What do they notice happens when they practice noticing those parts?
5. Alternate rounds between observing the external environment and noticing internal experiences. Encourage the client to continue practicing this game at home.

Affirmations List

Therapeutic Rationale

This activity invites kids to develop a list of affirmations—kind, supportive phrases that remind them of their personal strengths and who they really are. In ACT, affirmations aren't about avoiding discomfort or pretending everything is okay, but about offering grounded, present-moment support. From the lens of self-as-context, affirmations help kids speak from the perspective of the observing self—the part of them that notices thoughts and feelings without being defined by them.

Goals

- Reinforce the idea that the self is bigger than any single thought or feeling
- Support mindful reflection and self-compassion
- Build a personalized toolbox of affirming phrases

Materials

- Blank paper
- Writing utensil

Instructions

1. Explain to the client that affirmations are kind, truthful reminders we can give ourselves. They don't erase uncomfortable thoughts or feelings, but they help us make space for those feelings without being overwhelmed by them. Emphasize that the client can use affirmations to remember who they are and what they care about.
2. To help your client create their own affirmations, offer some reflection prompts:
    - "What do you want to remember about yourself on a tough day?"
    - "What words do you wish someone else would say to you?"
    - "What's something you believe is true about yourself no matter what?"
    - "What's something that helps you feel brave, strong, or loved?"
    - "What would your favorite person or character say to lift you up?"
3. Encourage clients to write 5 to 10 affirmations. Examples include:
    - "I am doing my best, and that is enough."
    - "Thoughts are just thoughts. They don't control me."
    - "I am learning and growing."
    - "I am more than any one moment."
    - "It's okay to be a work in progress."

- "I matter, even when things feel hard."
- "I can feel scared and still move forward."

4. Invite the client to keep the list by their bed, in a school folder, or on their mirror. They can read the list once daily, choose one to repeat when feeling overwhelmed, or pick a "daily affirmation" to carry with them.

Me Tree

Therapeutic Rationale

Children, like trees, grow, change, and face challenges, but they also have the ability to choose what nourishes them. In this activity, clients imagine themselves as a tree—where the trunk and branches represent their values and strengths, and the leaves are their thoughts and feelings that come and go. Just like leaves, thoughts and feelings can change or fall away, but the trunk—the observing self, or self-as-context—remains steady and grounded. This perspective helps kids notice their experiences without being defined by them. Given that this exercise focuses heavily on values, it is most effective when done in conjunction with the values clarification exercises in Section 5: Values.

Goals

- Strengthen and internalize a deeply held concept of self
- Notice thoughts and feelings without fusing with them

Materials

- *Me Tree* template
- *Leaves* template
- Writing utensil
- Scissors
- Crayons, markers, or colored pencils

Instructions

1. Once your client has a sense of their values and attributes, introduce them to the Me Tree. Explain that this tree is made of powerful wood that can withstand anything. Its trunk and branches represent the client's strengths, values, and qualities that help them stand tall. Have them decorate and label the trunk and branches on the *Me Tree* template with these qualities.
2. Once they're done, ask your client if they notice anything peculiar about the tree. They should notice pretty quickly that it has no leaves! Explain that you are going to put the leaves on the tree yourselves, because of course trees need leaves!
3. Provide the client with a variety of blank leaves from the *Leaves* template (precut them before session or have the client cut them out) and ask them to write one thought or feeling per leaf that describe them. Encourage a mix of helpful, unhelpful, and neutral thoughts and feelings.
4. Discuss how leaves, like thoughts and feelings, can be pretty and full of life, ugly and dying, or somewhere in between. Eventually, though, all leaves fall, blow away, and are replaced by other leaves. In much the same way, if we let them, all of our thoughts and feelings will eventually fall and be blown away, lost in the wind. Regardless of the leaves, the tree itself always stands tall.

5. Invite your client to color each leaf with green for helpful thoughts and feelings and orange/yellow/brown for unhelpful thoughts and feelings. The goal is to make the less helpful leaves look unhealthy. Once each leaf is colored, have your client place it on their Me Tree.
6. Now invite your client to prune the tree by removing the unhealthy leaves. They can pluck the leaf off, blow it away, and watch it flutter to the ground. Anything that helps them remove the leaf!
7. Discuss what it feels like to release these leaves. If necessary, give them an opportunity to replace some of the dead leaves with new, healthier leaves.

Me Tree Template

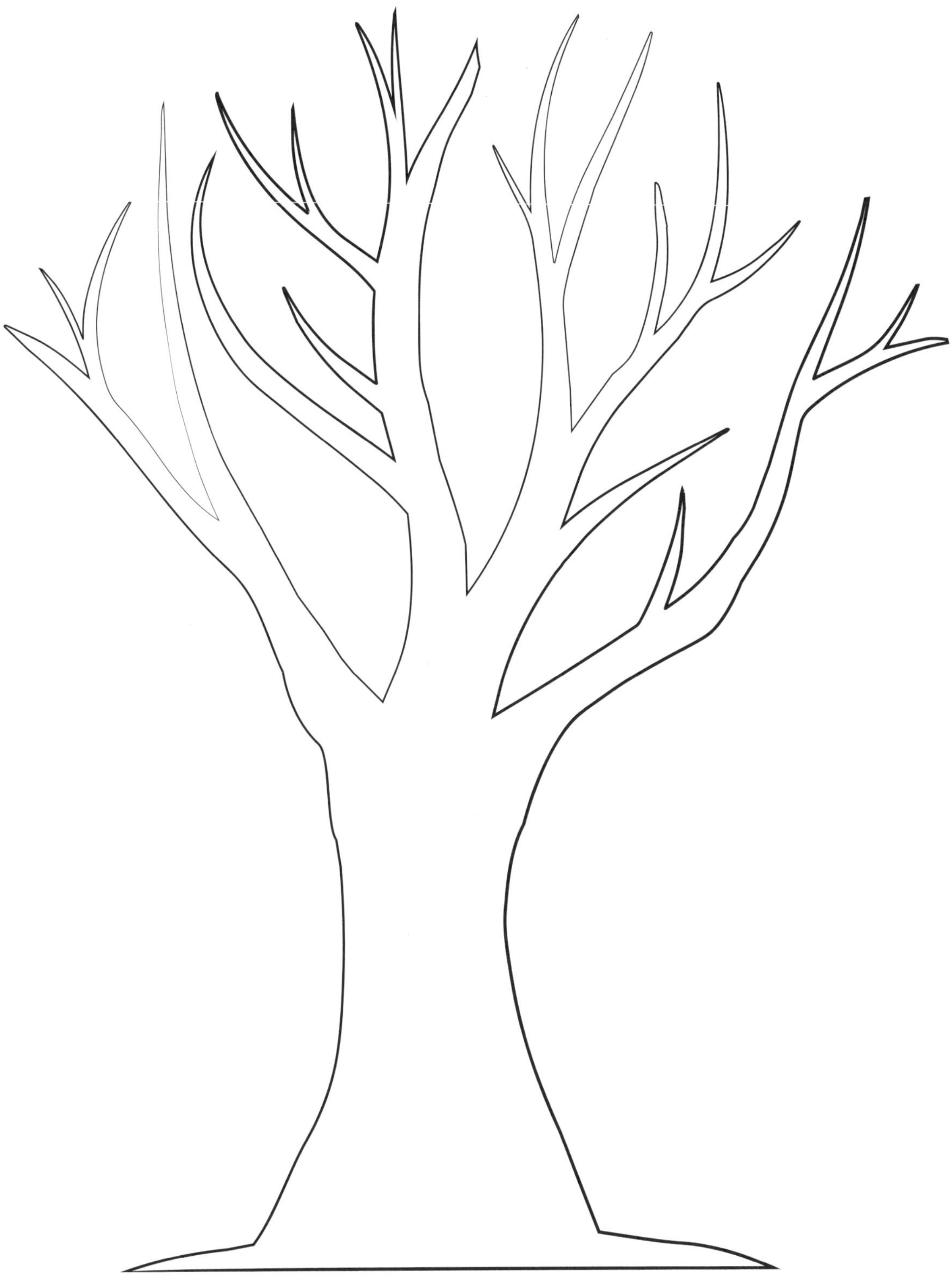

Leaves Template

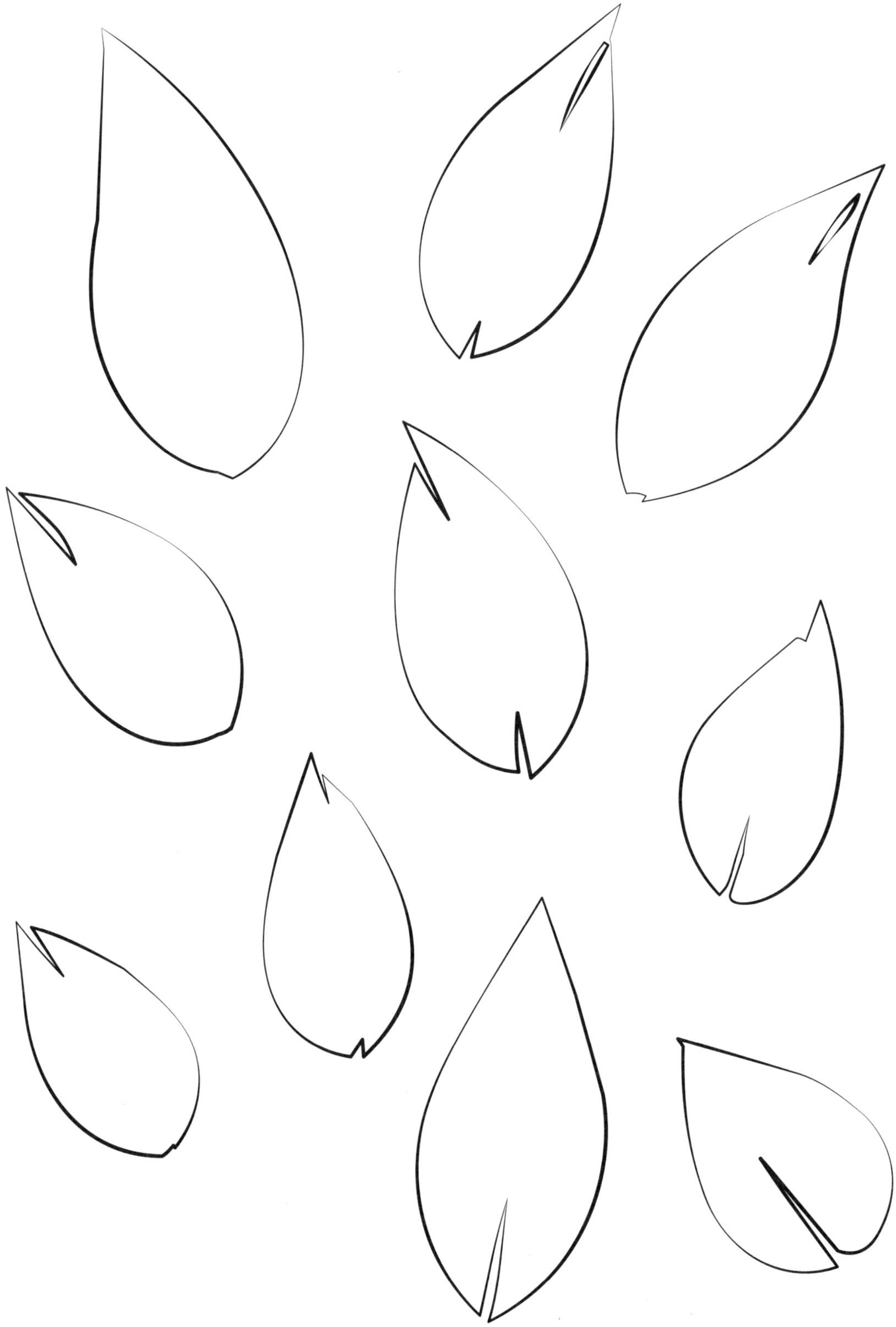

Notice Yourself Noticing

Therapeutic Rationale

While writing this book, Matt had an epiphany: He realized he was a grownup, with his own money, car, and the freedom to spend as he wished! Naturally, he went and bought himself a new video game system—and he realized something else: Video games are all about noticing. You notice your character's health level, hidden items, paths on the game map, and the environment around you. This makes it a perfect metaphor for kids to notice aspects of themselves and their life. Just as a gamer must observe without getting lost in every detail, kids can learn to notice their thoughts and feelings without being caught up by them.

Goals

- Practice cognitive defusion with regard to self-as-context
- Combine self-as-context skills with mindfulness

Materials

- *Noticing Log* worksheet

Instructions

1. Invite your client to share some of their favorite video games. Have a brief conversation about this, both to gain context and to build rapport. Self-disclosure may also be appropriate here. Do you love playing *Madden* or *Fortnite*? Tell them!
2. Ask your client if every video game looks the same. Are they always observing from a first-person perspective? Or a third-person perspective? Of course not! Different video games require different perspectives.
3. Remind your client that no matter what kind of video game they play, they usually have to track multiple things simultaneously—timers, health meters, powerups, boss fights, and the like. It's a lot to balance! Ask them how they do so successfully.
4. Explain that this ability to notice and track multiple things at once is a skill—and it's a skill they can use in life too. That skill is called "noticing."
5. Discuss that the *real* skill is to notice ourselves noticing. We can notice all sorts of things without becoming overly distressed or excited by them. For example, in a video game, we can notice that there are only a few seconds left to beat the level, notice how we feel inside as the timer ticks down, and notice how good it feels to beat the level.
6. Ask your client to think of other times in their life it may be helpful to practice noticing. Brainstorm ideas with them.
7. For homework, assign them the *Noticing Log* worksheet. Have them record what they notice simultaneously in the external world (e.g., colors, sounds, people) and in their

internal world (e.g., thoughts, feelings, body sensations), using the example in the log as a model. In the next session, discuss whether noticing helped them respond rather than react (e.g., by allowing them to regulate their emotions, choose to take committed action, and so on).

Noticing Log Worksheet

Each day, notice one thing in the world around you (external) and one thing inside yourself (internal) at the same time.

Date	External Noticing (What You See and Hear)	Internal Noticing (What You Feel and Think)
8/15	Kids laughing on the bus ride to school	Nervous about my science test

SECTION 5

Values

When you ask someone if they know what their values are, they usually say, "Of course! What kind of a silly question is that?" They scoff . . . until you ask them to actually name them. "Um, well . . . one value is . . . um . . . is wanting pizza a value? I like pizza."

Values are ideas that we know and feel deeply to be true to us, yet many people (especially kids) can struggle to put them into words. Part of the problem is that we often mix up values with goals. Goals are things we can accomplish and check off a list; once they are done, they stay done. "Buying a house," "graduating from school," or "starting a family" are all goals. Values, on the other hand, are aspirational. They are never done. Nobody wakes up one day and says "Yay! I've finally accomplished kindness. I can check it off the list and go rob banks now."

Both goals and values are important in our lives, but research has consistently shown that engaging in committed action in pursuit of meaningful values tends to lead to greater fulfillment and contentment with life. It does not even particularly matter what those values are. Someone who cherishes and pursues "love" is not inherently happier than someone who pursues "independence." What matters is that those values are truly meaningful to the individual—and that they pursue them.

This is not to say that living according to one's values guarantees constant happiness. That's not the point. Kids will still experience frustration, sadness, anxiety and disappointment. The goal is not to eliminate uncomfortable emotions, but to help kids feel content and satisfied with the direction in which they are steering the ship of their lives. If kids can truly do that, then it almost doesn't matter how they feel in a given moment. Good, bad, happy, sad . . . these are temporary states of being. But contentment and fulfillment persevere and transcend. And one way to help kids cultivate values is by doing values-based work.

Values Foundations

Therapeutic Rationale

This activity is designed to help kids identify their values and put them into words. Values are the things that truly matter to a child: the kind of person they want to be, the ways they want to treat others, and what they want their life to stand for. Using the compass analogy, this activity teaches kids that values help guide the direction of their choices, even though they do not tell them exactly what to do. While goals can be completed, values are ongoing and lived out over time, providing the foundation for later values-based work in therapy.

Goals

- Introduce concept of values
- Differentiate between values and goals

Materials

- *Values Foundation* worksheet
- Writing utensil

Instructions

1. Introduce the concept of values: "Values are like a compass. They don't tell us exactly *where* to go, but they help us choose the *direction* we want to move in."
2. Share the difference between values and goals: "Values and goals are both equally important, but they are not the same. A goal can be completed (like getting a good grade on a math test), but a value is ongoing (like caring about getting an education). We never 'finish' being a kind person or 'complete' being a loyal friend; we just keep living in that direction."
3. Explain that values, while never ending, can change and adapt over time. Just like people grow and change, values can too. Some values stay important throughout a person's life, while others become more or less important over time. What matters to someone at age 8 might very well change at ages 18 and 38, and that is okay!
4. Use the following questions to help your client start thinking about what matters to them. There are no wrong answers!
    a. "What do you care deeply about?"
    b. "When do you feel the most *yourself*?"
    c. "Who do you look up to and why?"
    d. "If you could be known for something, what would it be?"
    e. "What makes a 'good day' feel good?"
    f. "If your values were a compass, which direction are you facing right now? Are you moving in the direction of the things that matter most?"
5. Provide the *Values Foundation* worksheet to help the client identify potential values that resonate with them. They can circle the values that are important to them on the handout or include their own examples.

Values Foundation Worksheet

Achievement	Love
Adventure	Loyalty
Athleticism	Morals
Being a good student	Musicality
Being silly	Peace
Bravery	Power
Calmness	Religion
Creativity	Responsibility
Family	Safety
Fairness	Spirituality
Fame	Sportsmanship
Friendship	Stability
Fun	Success
Freedom	Teamwork
Helping others	Trying your best
Honesty	Variety
Humor	Wealth
Kindness	Winning
Leadership	

Give and Take

Therapeutic Rationale

Kiddos often struggle to understand family systems from a perspective other than their own. They may feel frustrated because they believe they are doing *so much more* than anyone else in their family, or because they feel like it should not be their responsibility to contribute at all. This activity helps kids recognize that everyone in a family has different roles and responsibilities.

Goals

- Facilitate understanding and empathy regarding familial roles
- Instill a sense of personal responsibility

Materials

- *Give and Take* worksheet
- Writing utensil

Instructions

1. Begin by asking your client what a family is. Their answers may vary, but guide the conversation toward the idea that a family is a group of people who care about each other, and that in a family, everyone both contributes to and receives support from the group.
2. Ask your client if they believe that everyone in a family has the same job. Most children will say no, which is correct—roles differentiate based on age, ability, and developmental level. For example, it would be weird for a parent to go to school while a child goes to work!
3. Explain that you want to think about the child's roles in their family. Together, fill out the *Give and Take* worksheet. Under the "give" column, include their contributions, like going to school and helping with chores. Under the "take" column, list the necessities and supports they receive, like food, water, shelter, clothing, love, and safety.
4. Once the worksheet is complete, offer some reflection prompts:
    a. "How do you feel about the ratio of give to take?"
    b. "How well do you fulfill the items under 'give'?"
    c. "Do you feel like the distribution is fair?"
5. Be sure to nonjudgmentally point out any incongruities between what the child says (e.g., "I do all the chores") versus what actually occurs (e.g., they only do some chores).
6. Ask your client what they may want to change, either in what they give or what they take.
7. As an extension, family members can complete their own lists and share them together. How does each person feel about each other's lists? Would anyone want to change anything? What happens when someone doesn't live up to their "give" responsibilities?

Give and Take Worksheet

Describe what you *give* to your family (things you do or contribute) and what you *take* from your family (things you receive or need).

Give	Take

Skill Practice and Application

Inside Me, Outside Me

Therapeutic Rationale

Children often feel intense guilt or shame about their thoughts, emotions, and urges. However, thoughts, emotions, and urges have no direct bearing on the world or other people—only actions do. This activity helps kids identify the difference between internal experiences and external actions, reinforcing the idea that having a thought or urge that conflicts with their values does not make them a bad person.

Goals

- Differentiate between internal experiences and external actions
- Reduce guilt or shame related to internal experiences
- Encourage values-driven actions regardless of incongruent internal experiences

Materials

- *Inside Me, Outside Me* worksheet
- Writing utensil

Instructions

1. Introduce this activity after a client reports feeling guilt or shame related to an internal experience. Ask if they feel guilt, shame, or both. You may need to provide psychoeducation on the difference: Guilt is feeling bad about something we've *done*, while shame is feeling bad about something we believe we *are*.
2. Ask your client to consider the following: "What if I told you that you don't have to feel guilt or shame about that thought? In fact, what if I told you that you don't have to feel guilt or shame about *any* thought?" Explore their reaction to this idea, including any resistance.
3. Explain that guilt and shame are not appropriate responses to thoughts, urges, or feelings because these are entirely internal experiences. They only occur entirely in the brain and have no impact on the world at large. If something does not affect others, it cannot have any moral value—positive or negative—and therefore guilt or shame is not warranted.
4. It may take your client some time to process this idea, so answer their questions and provide support as needed.
5. Introduce the *Inside Me, Outside Me* worksheet to help your client differentiate between thoughts, emotions, urges, and actions. Use the worksheet to revisit the recent internal experience that triggered guilt or shame. Together, classify the experience: Is it a thought, feeling, urge, or action? Does the experience happen inside them or outside them? Is guilt or shame an appropriate response? Why or why not?

Inside Me, Outside Me Worksheet

Think about something that recently made you feel guilty or ashamed. Fill out the following chart to describe that experience. For each row, describe: (1) what the experience was, (2) whether it's a thought, feeling, urge, or action, (3) whether it happened inside you (thought, feeling, urge) or outside you (action), and (4) whether it would make sense to feel guilty or ashamed.

Experience	Is It a Thought, Feeling, Urge, or Action?	Is It Inside Me or Outside Me?	Is Guilt or Shame Appropriate?
I wanted to hit my sister.	Urge	Inside	No
I stole my brother's toy.	Action	Outside	Yes

Using Values to Build Goals

Therapeutic Rationale

This activity helps kids understand the difference between values and goals, and how linking the two can create more meaningful and sustainable action. Values are ongoing qualities of action—ways of being that guide how we want to show up in the world. Goals are specific, measurable steps we take along the way. When kids learn to anchor their goals in their values, they are more resilient when setbacks arise and more intrinsically motivated to persist even through discomfort.

This activity is particularly helpful early into the therapeutic relationship so that you and your client can clarify the direction of your work together. Values-based goals can, and should, be revisited and revised over time as goals are met or change.

Goals

- Identify goals grounded in personally meaningful values
- Promote awareness that values-based action feels purposeful and fulfilling

Materials

- *Using Values to Build Goals* worksheet
- Writing utensil
- *Values Foundation* worksheet (optional)

Instructions

1. Begin by reviewing the concept of values and ask the client to list a few that are important to them. You can return to the *Values Foundation* worksheet on page 198 if needed.
2. Remind the client that values, like a compass, help point us in the direction of our goals. Explain that today they'll identify goals that are guided by their values "compass" so they can connect what matters most to them to the actions they can take.
3. Introduce the *Using Values to Build Goals* worksheet and work through the columns together:
    a. **Goal I want to work on:** Ask the client to write a goal that feels meaningful to them. Encourage them to think about something they want to improve or achieve in a way that connects to their values.
    b. **Values that will help me work toward it:** Help the client identify two to four values that will guide their actions toward this goal. Discuss how each value connects to the goal.
    c. **Steps to help me get there:** Break the goal into specific, concrete, and measurable steps. Encourage the client to think about what they can do daily, weekly, or monthly to work toward the goal. Use small steps first to build confidence.
4. Revisit the worksheet regularly, adjusting goals or steps as needed.

Using Values to Build Goals Worksheet

Use this worksheet to turn your important values into a goal and identify the steps you can take to work toward that goal.

Goal I Want to Work On	Values That Will Help Me Work Toward It	Steps to Help Me Get There
Build a better relationship with my family by reducing fights about my messy room	Family, responsibility, kindness, love	1. Clean my room 2 minutes every day before bed 2. Spend 20 minutes once a week doing extra tidying up 3. Once a month, do a deep clean for 1 hour

Bravery Ladder

Therapeutic Rationale

In ACT, exposure is not about "getting over" anxiety or fear. It's about building a life that matters by moving through difficult situations while bringing fear and anxiety along for the ride. Unlike traditional exposure ladders that focus on reducing distress, an ACT-based bravery ladder helps clients work toward meaningful goals, even in the face of discomfort. To support this idea, this activity introduces the concepts of willingness and values-based action—the idea that we can feel scared *and* take steps toward what matters. It also shows that even slow, sometimes small, steps help us progress toward our goals.

Goals

- Reframe exposure as values-based action, not symptom elimination
- Emphasize that meaningful action can happen even in the presence of fear or anxiety
- Build confidence through small, measurable acts of bravery

Materials

- *Bravery Ladder* worksheet
- Writing utensil

Instructions

1. Introduce the concepts of willingness and values-based action. Explain that we don't need to eliminate our fears to move toward what matters to us; we just learn to carry the fear with us. It may make sense to show a short movie clip or reference a character your client admires who does something brave *while* feeling scared.
2. Ask questions to explore the client's fear and avoidance:
   a. "What is something that makes you nervous or anxious?"
   b. "Does this worry ever hold you back or get in the way of something you care about?"
   c. "What does it mean to be brave?"
   d. "What does bravery look like for you?"
3. Help the client to identify a goal that matters to them—something they want to do but avoid because of fear or anxiety. It should be something you can help them break down into clear, manageable steps, like giving a presentation in front of the class.
4. Start building their exposure hierarchy by putting this meaningful goal at the top of the *Bravery Ladder* worksheet. Then work backward by identifying smaller substeps that build toward that goal. For example, before presenting in class, the steps might include

rehearsing lines at home, practicing with a family member, answering a question in class, and practicing the full presentation with a peer. The important part is that these are things the client can measure and work toward.

5. Remind the client that the goal is *not* to make the fear go away, but to become more flexible at handling it. Reinforce that every step on the ladder is an act of courage and not a test of fearlessness. They can do hard things, even when it feels scary!

Bravery Ladder Worksheet

Write your main goal at the top of the ladder, then break it down into smaller steps, with each rung of the ladder representing an action that brings you closer to that goal.

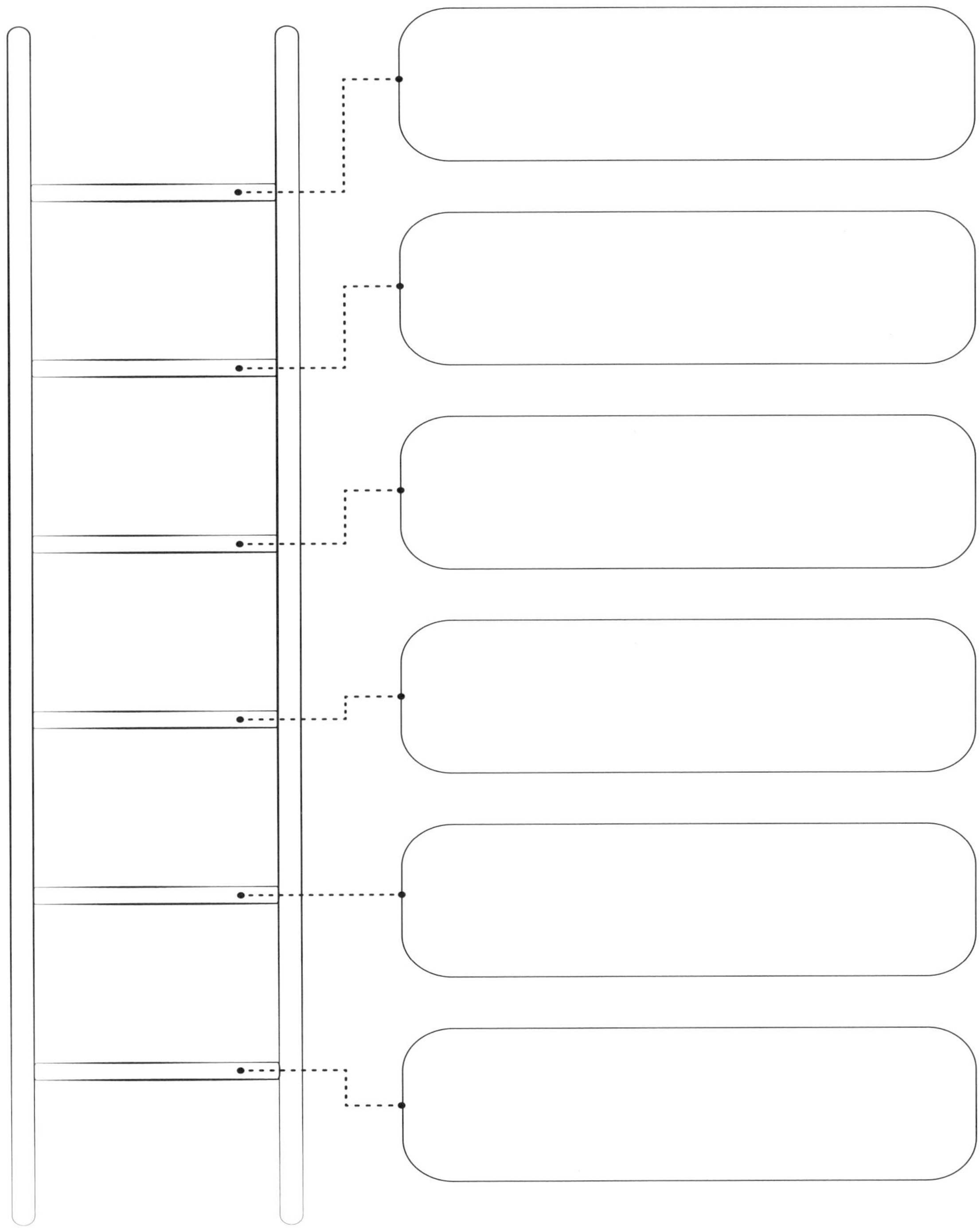

Values Spectrum

Therapeutic Rationale

This activity builds on the *Healthiness Spectrum* activity on page 56 in Section 2: Cognitive Defusion. It has been adapted to explore how actions align (or don't align) with a child's stated values. By visualizing choices on a spectrum, kids can reflect on whether their actions move them closer to or farther away from the life they want to lead. This activity is best used when a child has identified actions that may be incongruent with their stated values.

Goals

- Strengthen and deepen earlier skills when it comes to decision-making
- Provide a practical framework to explore values-based action

Materials

- *Values Spectrum* handout
- *Healthiness Spectrum* handout

Instructions

1. Begin by reviewing the *Healthiness Spectrum* handout, and ask your client what they remember about it. Provide a brief refresher on its use and purpose.
2. Shift the focus from healthiness to values: Explore how the client's current values relate to the choices they are making. For example, helping a friend in need might move them closer to their values of kindness, while skipping chores might move them farther away from their value of responsibility.
3. Using the *Values Spectrum* handout, have your client reflect upon where their actions fall on the spectrum:
    a. Are they satisfied with the choices they are making?
    b. How are those choices moving them closer to or further from congruence with their stated values?
    c. If some actions are moving them farther away from their values, are they okay with that? If so, is it because they have two competing values and are prioritizing one over the other? Or is it because their stated value is not their actual value?
4. Work with your client to determine which actions they wish to adjust, add, or continue to move toward their stated values.
5. **Optional:** Examine the client's level of commitment to a given value on the spectrum. Do they expect perfection when it comes to living in accordance with this value? Do they allow themselves grace (or perhaps *too much* grace)? This promotes flexibility in values-based action.

Values Spectrum Handout

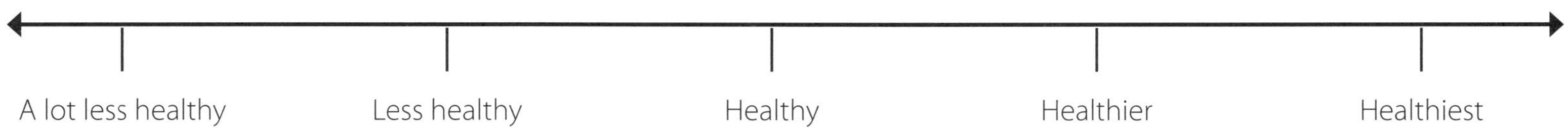

Skill Practice and Application

Family Values

Therapeutic Rationale

Family values reflect the shared principles and guiding beliefs that help a family navigate challenges, make decisions, and build stronger relationships. These values can grow and change over time, just like a child. In this activity, family members will reflect on what matters most to them, building mutual understanding and a shared language around expectations, behavior, and connection within the home.

Goals

- Create a shared language between children and caregivers
- Develop a set of family values for the home

Materials

- Blank paper
- Writing utensil
- Crayons, markers, or colored pencils
- Poster board
- *Values Foundation* worksheet (optional)

Instructions

1. Explain to the family that today they're going to think about what really matters to them as a family. What helps them grow, stay connected, and take care of each other, even when things get hard?
2. Give each family member a few minutes to quietly think about or write down answers to these questions:
   a. "What makes you feel most proud of your family?"
   b. "What do you do that makes your home feel safe or happy?"
   c. "What do you think is important about how you treat each other?"
   d. "What kind of people do you want to be—to each other and the world?"
3. Younger kids can draw pictures or pick from the examples on the *Values Foundation* worksheet (see page 198).
4. Invite each person to share what they wrote or drew. Are there any themes that show up more than once? Which ideas feel most important to each person? Are there any surprises?
5. Have the family work together to pick a few values they all agree on. There are no "right" answers—just what feels true and meaningful for the family. For example:
   - We value kindness. We treat others with respect, even when we disagree.
   - We value learning. We stay curious and try even when things are hard.
   - We value fun. We laugh and play together whenever we can.
6. Have the family write these down on a "family values" poster or frame them somewhere visible!

Skill Practice and Application

Stoplight Values

Therapeutic Rationale

Values are an inherently abstract concept to understand, which can make it difficult for kids to connect with their values and determine what is truly important to them. This activity uses a stoplight analogy to help kids to identify their values and explore how consistently those values are reflected in their current behaviors and choices.

Goals

- Identify the presence and absence of values in life
- Move toward values-based committed action

Materials

- *Stoplight Values* template
- Writing utensil
- Red, yellow, and green crayons, markers, or colored pencils

Instructions

1. Begin by clarifying the client's completed *Values Foundation* worksheet (see page 198) to help them reconnect with their identified values.
2. Explain that for this activity, they'll transfer their chosen values onto the *Stoplight Values* template and reflect on how each of those chosen values shows up in their everyday life through their actions and choices. They will decide whether each value belongs in the green, yellow, or red section of the stoplight and then color it accordingly.
    a. **Green:** This value is fully present in their life and reflected in their daily choices and behaviors.
    b. **Yellow:** The value is somewhat present in their life, but they want to take more actions to live this value consistently.
    c. **Red:** The value is minimally present or not present at all. Their daily choices and behaviors rarely align with this value.
3. Once the stoplight is complete, explore the results with the client. For the values that are marked in yellow or red, consider the following questions:
    a. What specific steps can they take to makes these values more present? For example, if kindness is their value, they might plan to help someone in need at least once per week.
    b. What obstacles are preventing this value from being more present? Is it lack of time, stress, conflicting values, or something else?
    c. What fears or worries do they have about making these changes?
4. Help the client develop a concrete action plan to increase the presence of their values. Revisit the stoplight in future sessions to track their progress. Are the colors the same, or have they changed? What strategies have helped? What barriers still remain?

Stoplight Values Template

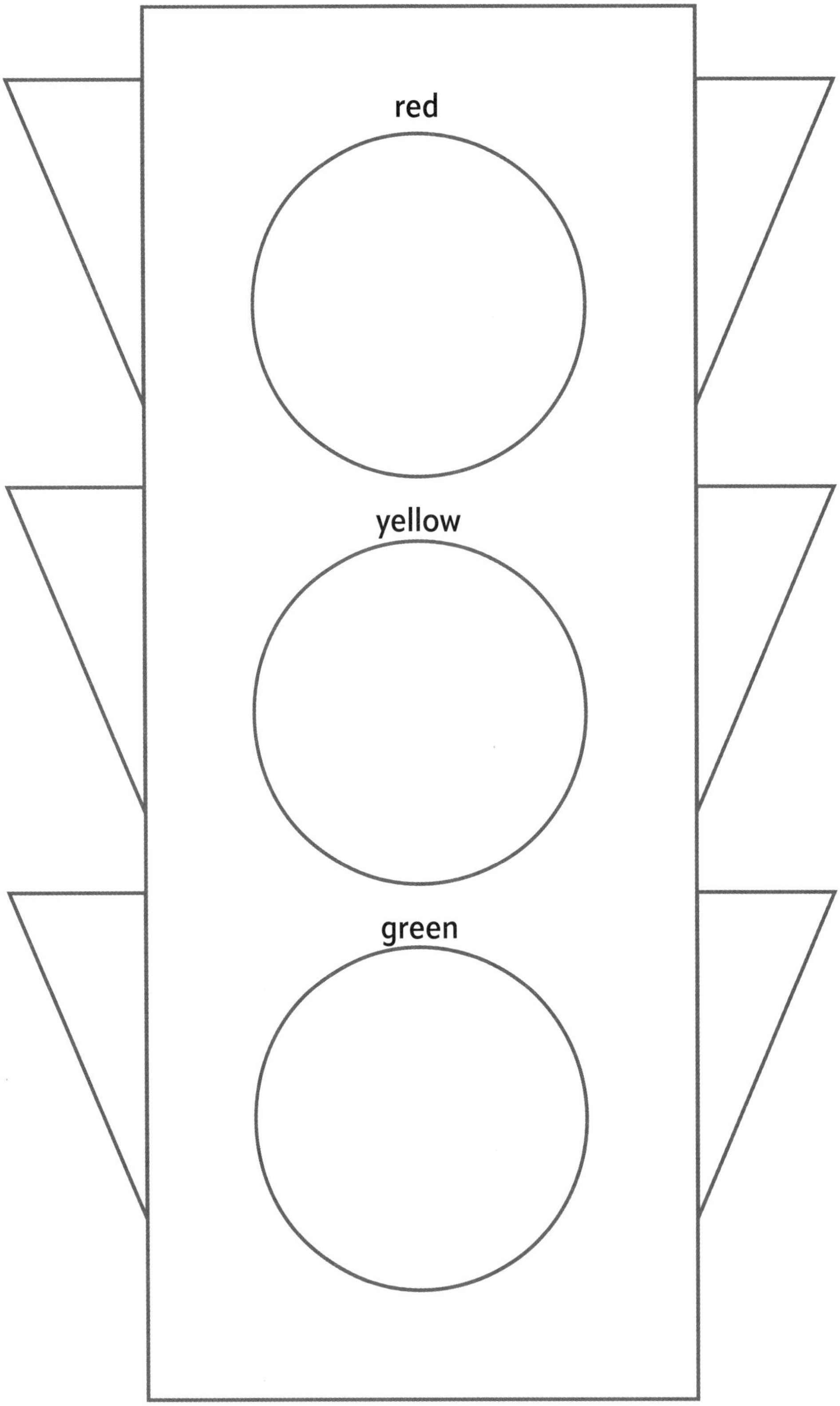

Values Venn Diagram

Therapeutic Rationale

This activity helps kids and their families begin to explore how their values align and differ. It supports the idea that even when people come from different backgrounds or seem very dissimilar, they often share underlying values that can help them understand each other, work together, and feel more connected. By mapping these values in a Venn diagram, kids can visually see where their values overlap and use that shared ground to set meaningful goals together.

Goals

- Increase awareness of personal and shared values
- Identify overlapping values that can support shared goals and improve communication

Materials

- *Values Venn Diagram* template
- *Values Foundation* worksheet
- Writing utensil

Instructions

1. After completing the previous *Values Foundation* worksheet with both the client and another family member (e.g., caregiver, sibling), have the client write down their personal values on one side of the Venn diagram, and the other participant write their values on the other side.
2. Ask them to look for values that overlap and write these shared values in the middle of the Venn diagram.
3. If they both care about a shared value—respect, for example—help the client notice that each person might express it differently: "It looks like you both value respect. What does respect mean to each of you? How do you show it?"
4. Notice the values that are unique to each individual. Invite them to share why those values are important to them and how they show up in their lives.
5. Collaboratively brainstorm ways to move forward with these shared values at the center of their relationship. How can they honor these values in their interaction, decisions, and routines?
6. Encourage them to keep the Venn diagram somewhere visible as a reminder of their shared values and as a prompt to keep moving toward their values.

Values Venn Diagram Template

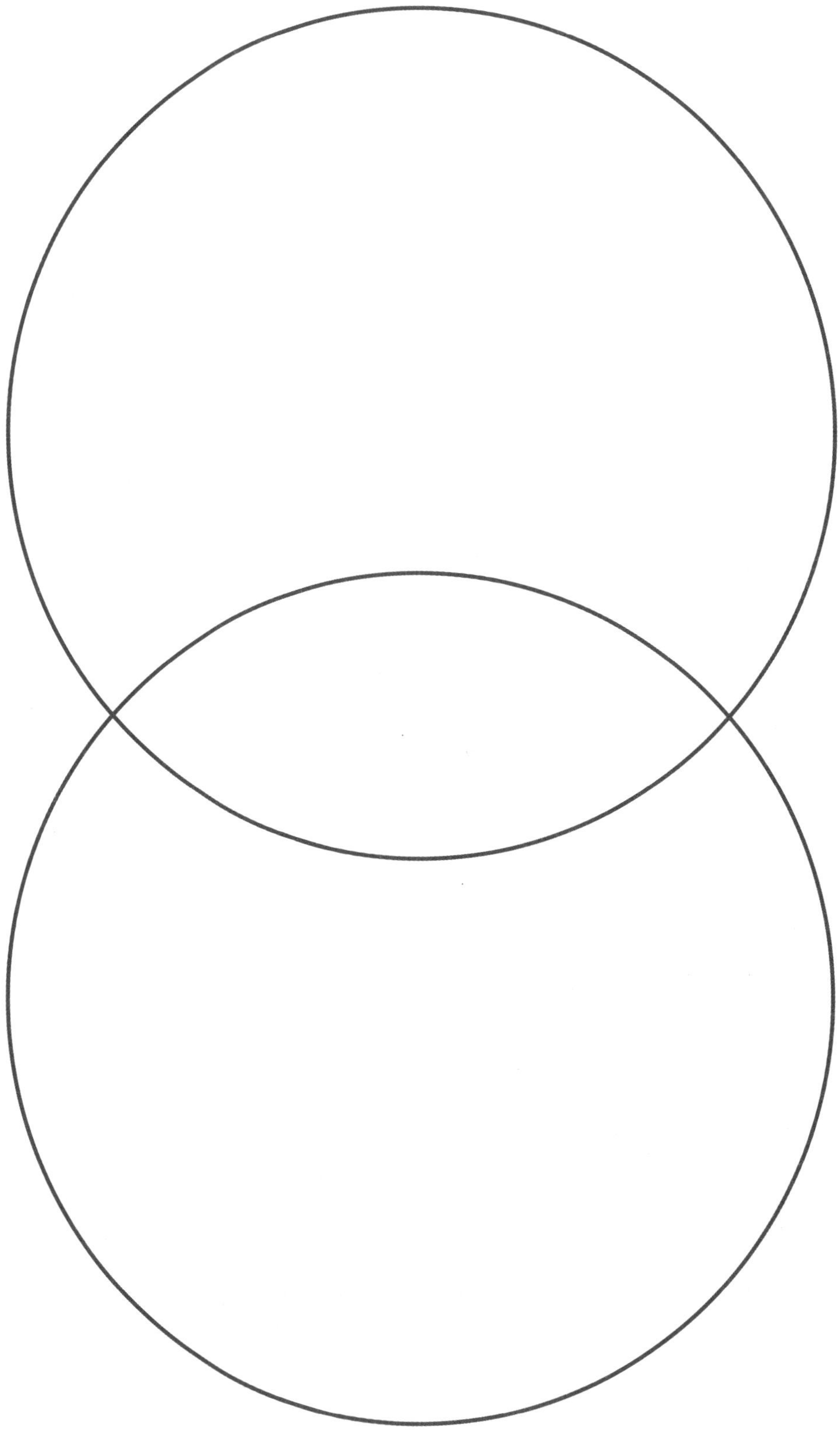

Value City

Therapeutic Rationale

This activity helps kids and families understand how our time, energy, and emotional space—represented by Monopoly game money—are limited resources. Spending them on what matters most (our values) can help feel more fulfilled and energized. By playing this adapted version of Monopoly, kids can see how their decisions, unexpected events, and other people's differing values can affect their ability to live by their own values.

Goals

- Build insight into values-driven decision-making
- Notice how emotional space is affected by unexpected events
- Reflect on how choices align with what truly matters

Materials

- Monopoly board game (we suggest the "junior" version for younger clients)
- Customized Chance cards (optional)

Instructions

1. Ask the client if they have ever played Monopoly. Ask what they liked about it, how they played before, and if they remember any of the rules. If they're new to the game, that's fine! Simply let them know you will be playing a different version today with a few new rules. If a caregiver or other adult is participating in session, invite them to play as well.
2. Set up the game as usual and have the client select their character piece.
3. Introduce the board by explaining that each location they can "buy" represents a value or coping skill. These are all things that require emotional energy (i.e., money).
4. As you hand out the money, explain that it represents how much emotional space they can devote to these areas. By using their emotional space wisely, they can "refill" their energy as they move around the board.
5. As players move around the board, they spend their energy (i.e., money) to collect values and coping skills.
    a. If a player lands on a coping skill or value they already own, they gain an extra $2 to signify that using a value or coping skill increases their capacity.
    b. If a player lands on someone else's value, they have to spend some of their energy (money).
    c. Each time a player passes "Go," they collect money as they continue moving in the direction of their values.

6. If players land on a Chance card, they need to take on an unexpected task. You can create customized Chance cards to reflect this, such as, "You had a fight with your friends. This costs you $3 of energy" or "You noticed your energy running low, so you used a coping skill and gained $5 in energy."
7. Encourage players to notice and be aware of their space so that they have room to handle the unexpected.
8. Please note that the game itself may bleed into additional sessions while other games may be completed in one! It can also be helpful, depending on the client's understanding and engagement with the activity, to expand this activity into a second session to further emphasize the idea.
9. For clients who really engage with this activity, it can be a fun homework assignment to have them teach the game to their family, which reinforces their understanding of values and provides an opportunity to apply these concepts in real-life situations.

Relationship Continuum: Part 1

Therapeutic Rationale

Many clients, particularly children and adolescents, are often distressed about what they believe others say or think about them. While this can sometimes be projection on their part, it can also indicate a skewed sense of self or a distorted understanding of how much weight others' opinions should have. This activity helps kids examine and revise their understanding of the role other people's perceptions should play in their lives.

Goals

- Identify the different roles that people play in a client's life
- Examine whether relationships align with personal values

Materials

- *Relationship Continuum* worksheet
- Writing utensil

Instructions

1. Ask your client how they know someone is a friend, an enemy, or another type of relationship. Discuss different categories of relationships that exist, such as friend, acquaintance, enemy, close friend, romantic partner, family (biological and chosen), and self.
2. Using the *Relationship Continuum* worksheet, have your client list qualities of each relationship. For example, a friend might be fun and trustworthy, an enemy might be unkind and hurtful, and a romantic partner might be affectionate and understanding. Remind them that different types of relationships can have similar qualities.
3. Next, have them place people from their life into the appropriate categories. Remind them that some people can change categories over time, and some people can also fit into multiple categories. For example, someone may be a part of their family of origin and also an enemy or close friend.
4. When you're done, ask the client what it was like for them to fill this out. What surprised them? Who belonged in a category that they didn't expect? Do they want to consider changing any relationships to move someone to a different category? Are they satisfied with the quantity and quality of relationships in each category?

Relationship Continuum Worksheet

What makes a friend a friend? An enemy an enemy? It can sometimes be hard to figure out what category someone fits into in your life. In the following table, list some of the qualities that describe people in each category. Then list people in your life who fit into these categories.

Relationship Type	Qualities	Examples
Friend		
Acquaintance		
Enemy		
Close friend		
Romantic partner		
Family		
Self		

Skill Practice and Application

Relationship Continuum: Part 2

Therapeutic Rationale

This is an extension and should only be done after completing the *Relationship Continuum: Part 1* exercise (see page 217). It helps kids think not just about who is in their lives, but how much influence or weight each relationship should carry. By visualizing relationships along a graph, kids can better understand how their own self-view matters compared to the opinion of others—and learn to prioritize relationships that align with their values.

Goals

- Identify the different roles that people play in a client's life
- Examine whether relationships align with personal values

Materials

- *Relationship Continuum* worksheet (completed)
- *Relationship Graph* worksheet
- Writing utensil

Instructions

1. After completing part 1 of this activity, explain that part 2 will help them think about how much influence each relationship should have in their life. Show them the x and y axes on the *Relationship Graph* worksheet, where the x-axis represents "how much each person's opinion matters" and the y-axis represents "how important they are to me."
2. Have your client plot each relationship category along the axes, considering how important each person is and how much their opinion matters. The goal is for them to create a roughly 45-degree line, starting with the following points:
    a. **Top right of the graph:** Self (most important and highest influence)
    b. **Bottom left of the graph:** Enemy (least important and lowest influence)
3. Have them fill in the remaining categories along the line where they feel appropriate.
4. Ask your client how they determined their placement choices. Emphasize that the self should be in the top right because their own opinion is the most important. Challenge any placements that seem off, such as rating themselves too low or giving certain categories too much weight.
5. Ask the client to reflect on whether they've been living in a way that is congruent with this graph. For example, have they prioritized their own values and self-concept? Have they disregarded the feedback of enemies?
6. If appropriate, have the client complete a second graph plotting the actual people in their life along the line. Process their placements and determine how they feel about everyone's position.

Relationship Graph Worksheet

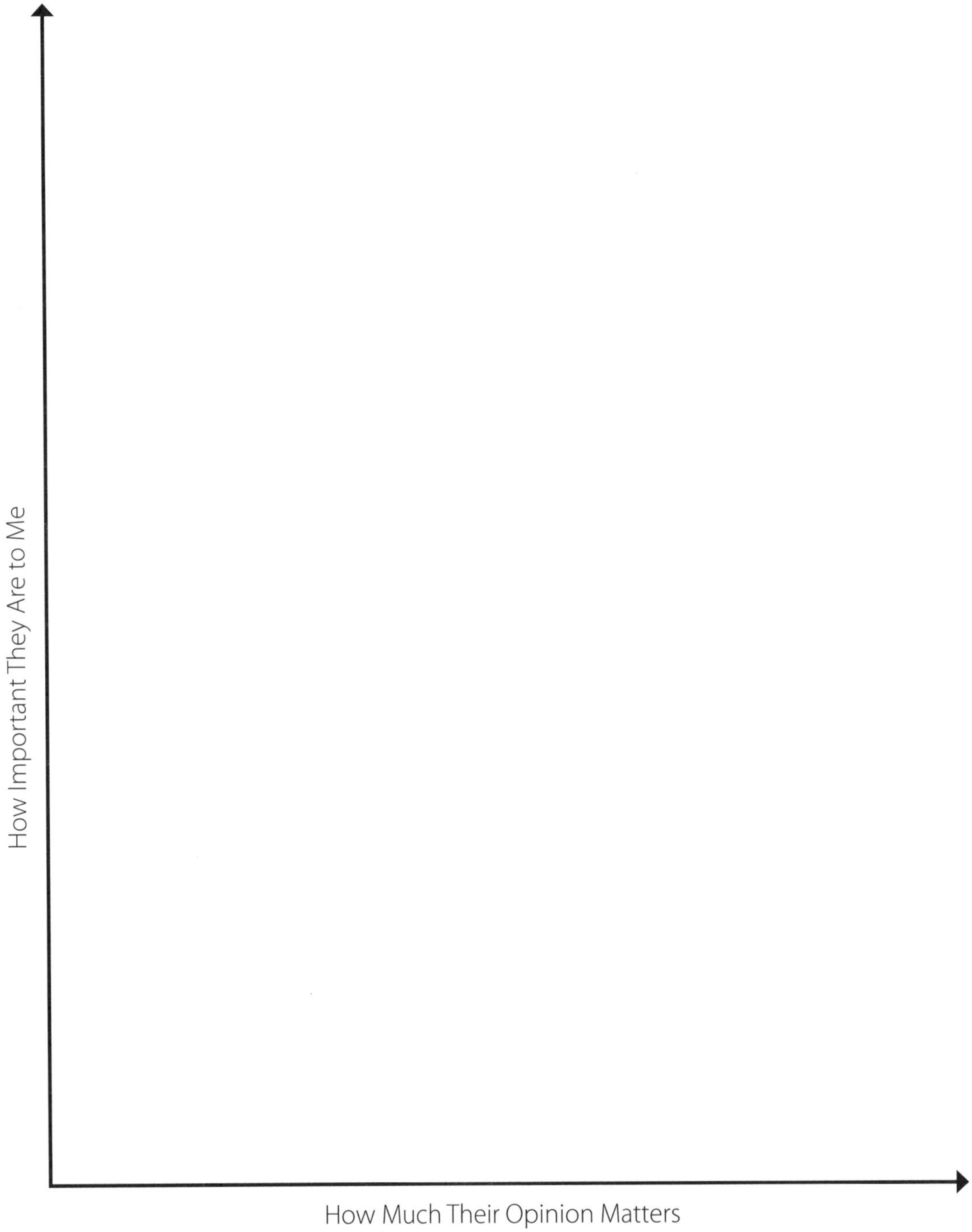

Skill Practice and Application

Filling Your Cup

Therapeutic Rationale

Relationships are inherently transactional. Some folks may find this to be a cold or cynical statement, but we promise it's not intended that way! What we mean is that relationships should provide benefit to both parties. Both people should be getting something out of a relationship. More to the point, both people should be able to get what they *need* from a relationship. This exercise is designed to help kids ensure that they are not dismissing their own wants and needs in a relationship in the name of being nice.

Goals

- Provide psychoeducation about healthy relationships
- Consider the roles that clients want others in their lives to fulfill

Materials

- *Filling Your Cup* worksheet
- Writing utensil

Instructions

1. Begin by sharing the metaphor of "filling your cup" with your client. Explain that it is impossible to take care of our own needs, much less help others, if our own cup is not full enough.
2. Continue the conversation by having your client identify activities and actions that fill their cup versus empty their cup. Note that some activities and actions can do both! For example, spending time with family and friends can be restorative while simultaneously requiring emotional energy and effort.
3. On the *Filling Your Cup* worksheet, have your client list some of their important relationships, as well as how those relationships add to or empty their cup. Encourage them to be honest, even if they don't love what they are writing.
4. Process their responses together. What do they feel about what they wrote? Are they satisfied with the balance of what fills their cup and what empties it? If not, what actions can they take so their relationships feel more balanced and fulfilling?

Filling Your Cup Worksheet

For each relationship you list, describe how it fills your cup (adds to your energy or happiness) and how it empties your cup (takes away energy or leaves you feeling drained).

Relationship	How It Fills My Cup	How It Empties My Cup

Cracks in the Sidewalk: Part 2

Therapeutic Rationale

This activity builds on part 1 of *Cracks in the Sidewalk* (see page 21). Part 1 introduced the concept of noticing emotional and cognitive "cracks" along the journey, whereas part 2 transitions into values-base response, where the child identifies and chooses to honor the values that guide them forward, even when the road isn't perfectly smooth. By turning the cracks into canvases, kids actively reframe challenges, pain, or discomfort into reminders of their purpose and the direction they want to move in.

Goals

- Connect everyday challenges with personal values
- Foster creativity and reflection by transforming emotional metaphors into visual, values-based reminders

Materials

- *Cracks in the Sidewalk: Part 1* worksheet (completed)
- Sidewalk chalk

Instructions

1. Begin by recapping part 1 of this activity. Revisit the idea that the "cracks" in the sidewalk—things like difficult memories, thoughts, or emotions—are always going to be part of the journey. While we can choose to turn around, we can also accept these cracks and continue down the road.
2. Explain that in this activity, the client will go beyond noticing the cracks and use them as reminders of what matters most to them—their values—so they can continue moving in in a forward direction.
3. If possible, go outside with the client during session or assign this as homework. Encourage them to use the chalk to write their values in the cracks, turning each challenge into a visual reminder of what matters most.
4. After they finish, process the activity together. Which values did they choose to write, and why? How did it feel to turn challenges into reminders of purpose? What did they learn about moving forward even when the road is difficult?

Values "Would You Rather?"

Therapeutic Rationale

Values can be a challenging concept for kids, particularly younger ones, to grasp. This activity uses the familiar and playful format of Would You Rather? questions to highlight what matters most to the child. By asking them to choose between two options, you can uncover what matters most and make the concept of values more accessible.

Goals

- Increase insight into personal values
- Support internal motivation by highlighting what is personally meaningful

Materials

- None

Instructions

1. Introduce the concept with a silly or lighthearted Would You Rather? question, such as "Would you rather have a pet lion or a pet whale?" Explain that by choosing, they highlight which option matters more to them. It's not that the other option isn't important, but they are just narrowing down what is most meaningful.
2. Go through the following list of questions and ask the client to go with their first instinct. You can also create additional customized questions based on your knowledge of the client or ask them to come up with some of their own:
    a. "Would you rather be right or kind?"
    b. "Would you rather be the bravest person in the room or the best problem solver?"
    c. "Would you rather win but damage a friendship or lose and gain a new friend?"
    d. "Would you rather be a great listener or a great storyteller?"
    e. "Would you rather stand up for someone you don't know or protect yourself?"
    f. "Would you rather be a great artist or a great athlete?"
    g. "Would you rather have super speed or invisibility?"
    h. "Would you rather be known for being funny or for being helpful?"
    i. "Would you rather take a risk or play it safe?"
    j. "Would you rather be good at math or good at reading?"
    k. "Would you rather have a lot of good friends or a few really good friends?"
    l. "Would you rather hang out with friends or family?"

3. If the client says, "Both are important," don't force a choice. Set both aside and revisit them later. If they remain unable to choose, discuss why each is important and what they mean to them.
4. Once complete, ask the client if they notice anything missing from the list. If so, be sure to add those too. Make a copy of their choices to reference in future sessions.

Values Card Sort

Therapeutic Rationale

To engage in committed action, kids need to know what values they are committing to. We have found that a card sort is a helpful way to introduce this concept because it provides a clear linguistic framework around which to explore their deeply held ideals. Many (if not most) kids feel their values intrinsically, but they often struggle to put them into words. This intervention accomplishes just that.

Goals

- Provide a linguistic framework to express values
- Explore, identify, and process values

Materials

- *Values Card Sort* template
- Blank note cards
- Writing utensil

Instructions

1. Provide your client with the *Values Card Sort* template. Explain that many (or most) of the cards may feel important to them in some way, but for this activity, they should choose the cards that are the *most* important. Do not give them a number to aim for. It is okay if they wind up with 20 or more cards! This is just the first step.
2. Once they've selected the first round, have them share their choices with you. Ask why they selected each card and how they narrowed down their selection.
3. Ask if anything important came to mind that wasn't on the cards. Examples might include being a good sibling or student. Allow the client to create a few new cards and add them to their stack.
4. Then, using only the cards they selected, have them repeat the exercise: "These are all important to you. Let's do it again—which are the most important?"
5. Process this second round in the same way, asking why they selected each card and how they narrowed their initial selection. Ask how it felt to discard previously selected cards.
6. Continue to repeat this process until they get down to approximately 5 to 8 cards. Ask the processing questions again, emphasizing how it felt to prioritize and discard cards, and how they feel about their top choices.
7. Conclude by discussing how values can change over time—and that is okay!—and that we're the most fulfilled when our values inform our goals. Work with your client to connect their top values to specific goals, either in their treatment plan, their life, or (ideally) both.

Values Card Sort Template

Adventure	Creativity
Asking for help	Curiosity
Athleticism	Emotional regulation
Being a good friend	Environmentalism
Being organized	Fairness
Being a problem solver	Flexibility

Being supportive	Forgiveness
Bravery	Fun
Caring for animals	Generosity
Calm	Gratitude
Compassion	Growth
Confidence	Helpfulness
Helping others	Playfulness

Humor	Power
Humility	Respect
Inclusion	Responsibility
Individuality	Safety
Justice	Self-care
Kindness	Self-control
Leadership	Seeing things through

Learning	Sharing
Learning from mistakes	Sportsmanship
Listening	Standing up for others
Loyalty	Teamwork
Patience	Thoughtfulness
Tolerance	Trying your best
Trust	Working hard

Confidence Compass

Therapeutic Rationale

This activity builds on the compass metaphor, illustrating that values, like a compass, lead us in the direction of our goals and the things that matter most. By filling in a compass with their personal values and supports—like coping skills, supportive people, or favorite activities—kids create a visual representation of what can guide them when they face challenges. This makes it easier to stay on the right path, make helpful choices, and keep moving toward their goals even in difficult situations.

Goals

- Create a visual representation of values
- Identify strategies to make it easier to move in the direction of values

Materials

- *Compass* template
- Writing utensil
- Crayons, markers, or colored pencils

Instructions

1. Introduce the *Compass* template and ask your client if they are familiar with a compass. If not, explain that a compass helps explorers know which direction to travel. Values work similarly, guiding us toward what matters most.
2. Ask the client to place their most important values around the compass. You can provide a preselected list of values they identified on the *Values Foundation* worksheet (see page 198), or let them come up with their own. Encourage them to think about what really matters to them, like honesty, kindness, or trying new things.
3. In the open spaces on the compass, have the client write things that help them stay on their path. This can include supportive people (e.g., friends, teachers), coping skills (e.g., deep breathing), or even favorite snacks or activities that motivate them!
4. Allow the client to decorate and personalize their compass with colors, drawings, or symbols that make it more meaningful and personal.
5. Encourage them to keep their compass in a visible place at home as a reminder of their values and the strategies they can use to navigate difficult situations.

Compass Template

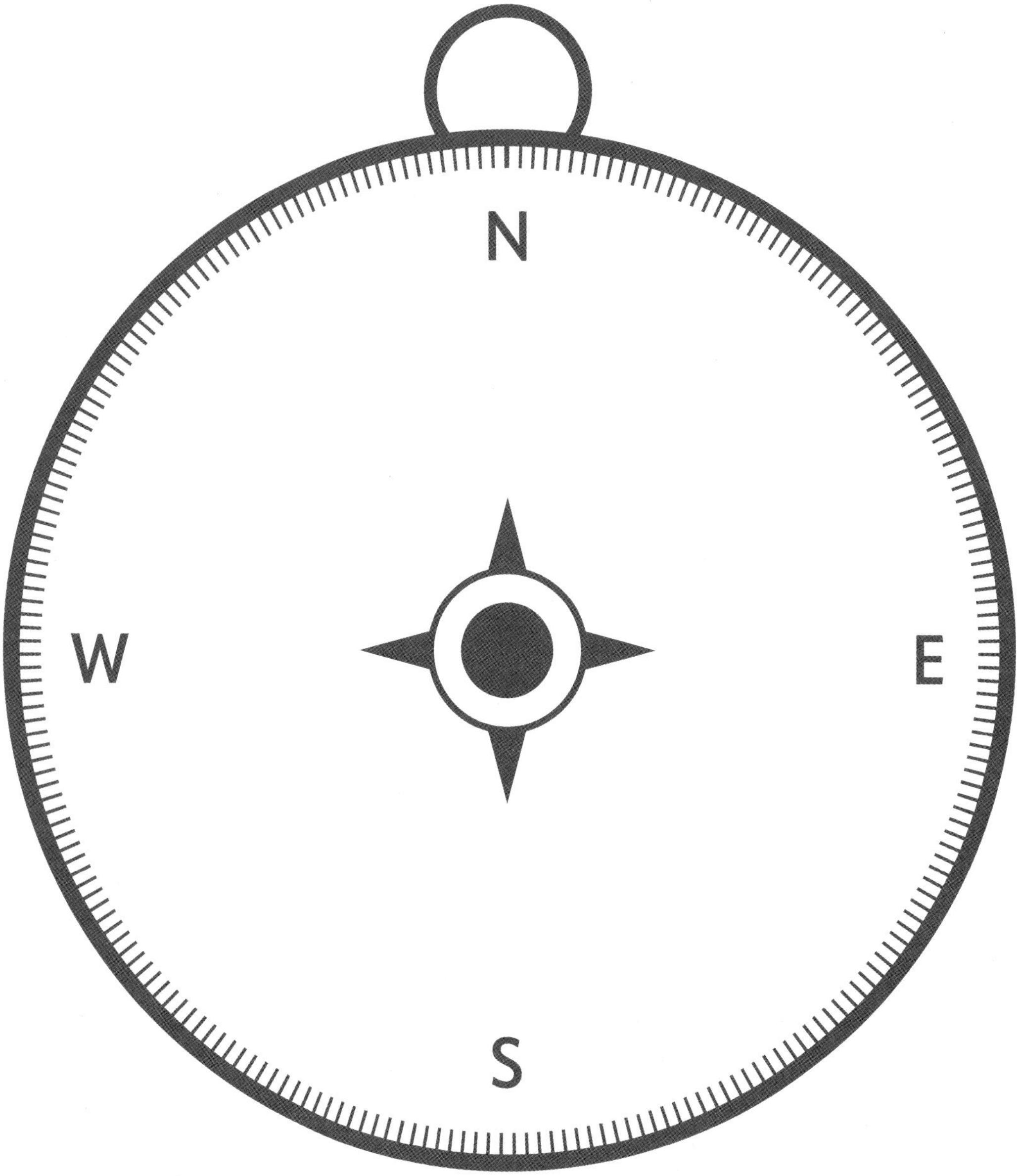

Weeding the Field

Therapeutic Rationale

Client: "I'm so mad at my friend. They did this, and they *know* how much it annoys me. I can't believe them."

Therapist: "What did they say when you talked with them about it?"

Client: "Uhh . . . I didn't."

We like joke to that our job as therapists would be unnecessary if people just talked to each other. So much distress, strife, and resentment grows, like weeds in a field, when we make assumptions or don't communication clearly. This activity is designed to help kids understand how unspoken expectations and miscommunication can "water the seeds" of resentment. It then invites them to practice "weeding the field" to make relationships healthier. It is most effective when a child has a specific concern or frustration rather than discussing the concept abstractly.

Goals

- Identify inaccurate assumptions that lead to resentment
- Approach conflict from a place of collaboration, not resentment or aggression

Materials

- *Field of Resentment* template
- Writing utensil

Instructions

1. Ask your client to share an upsetting interaction or relationship conflict they recently experienced, and ask what specifically about the interaction was distressing.
2. Explain that when people upset us, it's usually for one of two reasons: Either they don't know that something bothers us (ignorance), or they do know and choose to act that way anyway (malice). Emphasize that most of the time, people act out of ignorance rather than malice. For younger clients, frame this as "don't know" (ignorance) versus "don't care" (malice).
3. Ask whether they think the other person acted out of ignorance or malice. Explain that if they assume malice without having clearly communicated their wants or needs, it "waters the field" of resentment, making negative feelings grow.
4. Introduce the *Field of Resentment* template. Have the client write their feelings of resentment in the plants above the soil and the expectations they did not communicate in the roots below the soil. Explain that what we see above the ground is often fueled by what's happening underneath.

5. If the client says that the other person should have known what they wanted (or they believe they already did communicate clearly), explain that resentment is an indicator to slow down and double-check communication. Even when we think we've been clear, resentment often means expectations were still unspoken. Work with your client to strategize how they can be clearer about their needs using "I" statements.
6. Close the activity by brainstorming specific communication strategies they can use moving forward to "weed the field" and make resentment less likely to grow.

Field of Resentment Template

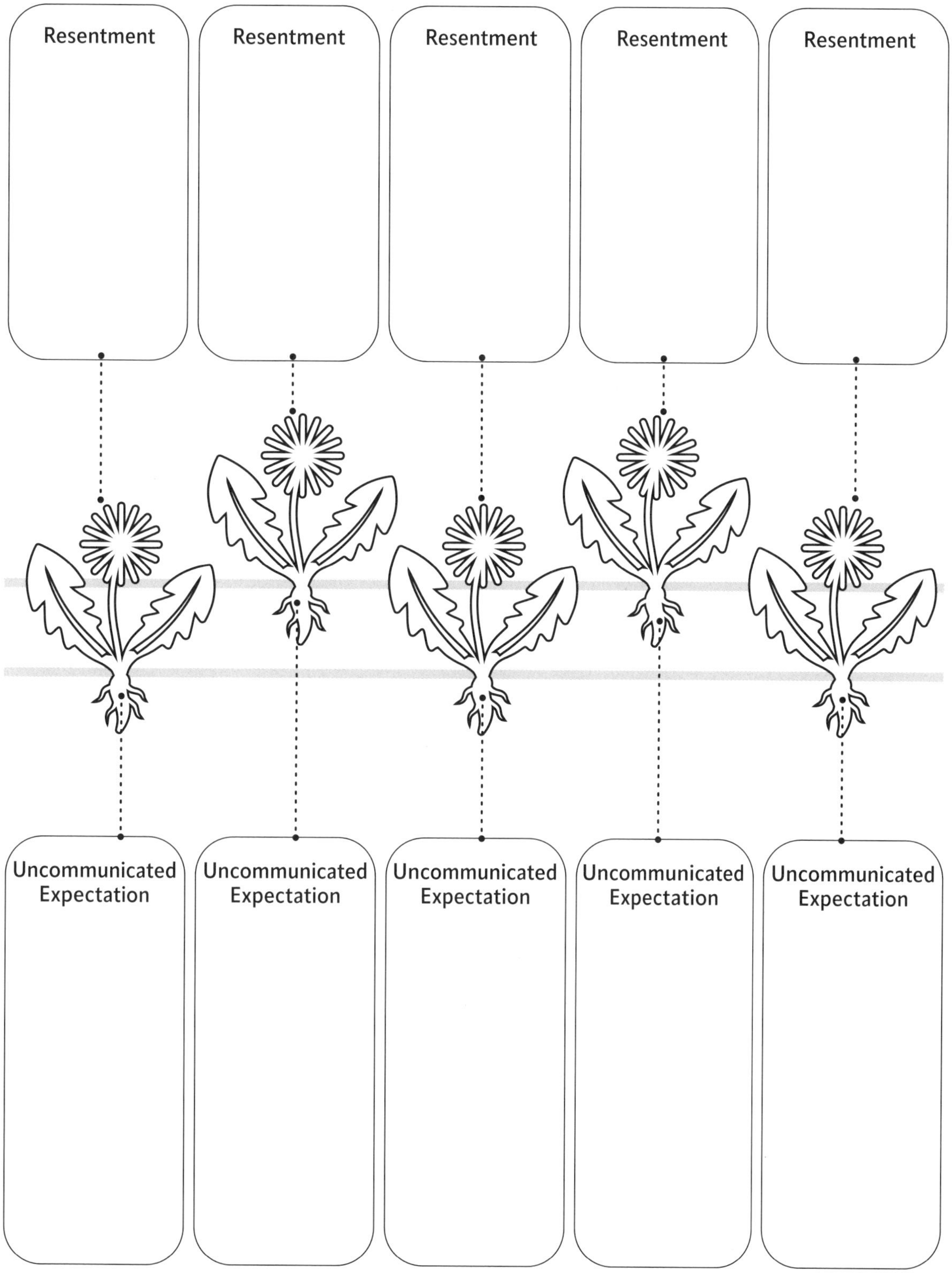

Ripples in the Water: Part 2

Therapeutic Rationale

Values guide how we want to live our lives, even when discomfort shows up along the way. In part 1 of this exercise (see page 169), we introduced the ripple metaphor to help kids visualize how different people, experiences, and ideas impact the "water" of their life. They identified these ripples and how close or far they were in relation to themselves. In part 2, kids will build on that work by exploring whether each ripple aligns with their values. They will also have the chance to think about how much influence they want to give to the ripples that *don't* align with their values moving forward.

Goals

- Examine the impact of people, events, thoughts, and emotions on the client's life
- Develop awareness of how those influences align with values

Materials

- *Ripples* template (completed)
- Writing utensil
- Red, yellow, and green crayons, markers, or colored pencils

Instructions

1. Begin by reviewing part 1 of this activity and notice who or what is represented in each ripple. If needed, create a new diagram to reflect any changes. Some ripples may have moved closer or farther away, or new ripples may have appeared.
2. Have the client identify whether each ripple aligns with their values. For example, a ripple might represent a supportive friend who encourages them be kind to others, which aligns with values like friendship and kindness. For the ripples that don't align with their values, discuss which values they conflict with and why. For example, a ripple might represent a peer who pressures them to lie or be mean, which goes against values like honesty and respect.
3. The client can use a color-coding system if they would like. For example, they can use green to represent ripples that align with values, yellow for ripples that sometimes align with values, and red for those that do not align with values. Using color makes it easier to see which ripples are supportive and which may need attention.
4. Ask the client to consider how much impact they want each ripple to have on their life. For example, they might want ripples from supportive friends, enjoyable activities, or positive memories to have a big impact, and ripples from stressful situations, upsetting memories, or uncomfortable emotions to have less influence. This can transition into a conversation about setting values-based goals regarding what to do and how to get there.

Sailing the Ship Toward Values Island

Therapeutic Rationale

The beauty of the hexaflex is that it is not hierarchical. The goal is not to figure out cognitive defusion completely, then figure out acceptance completely, and so on. The goal is to work on all six elements of the hexaflex simultaneously because each element nurtures and nourishes each other element. While this module is about values, values are worth very little without committed action based on those values. This intervention, which is inspired by Dr. Russ Harris,* is about incorporating both. It can be completed after some values exploration work has been done or serve as an introduction to values exploration.

Goals

- Turn values into committed action
- Incorporate multiple elements of the hexaflex simultaneously

Materials

- *Values Island* template
- Writing utensil
- Crayons, markers, or colored pencils

Instructions

1. Explain that today you will be talking about what really matters to your client—their values. Introduce the *Values Island* template and explain that the island on the right side is called "Values Island." This island represents the kind of person they want to be and the things that are most important to them in life.
2. Invite them to think about some of their most important values—for example, being kind, being honest, being a good friend, and so on. Have them write or draw these values in the blank spaces above Values Island.
3. Point out the ship on the left side of the coloring sheet and explain that the ship represents where they are right now. Explain that their goal is to sail to Values Island. It's a wonderful place, and when they make it there, they will feel content and at peace with life. However, to get there, they have to take committed actions to move the ship closer to the island, even when the ocean feels rough.
4. Work together to brainstorm actions that will help your client move their ship closer to Values Island. These actions should connect directly to their values—for example, "raise my hand in class" or "be honest even when it's hard." Have them write or draw these actions in the space between the ship and the island. Take some time with this! It should be an in-depth conversation.

---

* Russ Harris. (September 22, 2021). *Monsters on a boat* [Video]. YouTube. https://www.youtube.com/watch?v=vyxc889gQtY

5. To conclude the activity, have your client choose one or two committed actions they are willing to practice over the next week, and brainstorm a plan to perform those actions. Emphasize that success isn't about reaching the island right away, it's about continuing to steer the ship in that direction.

Values Island Template

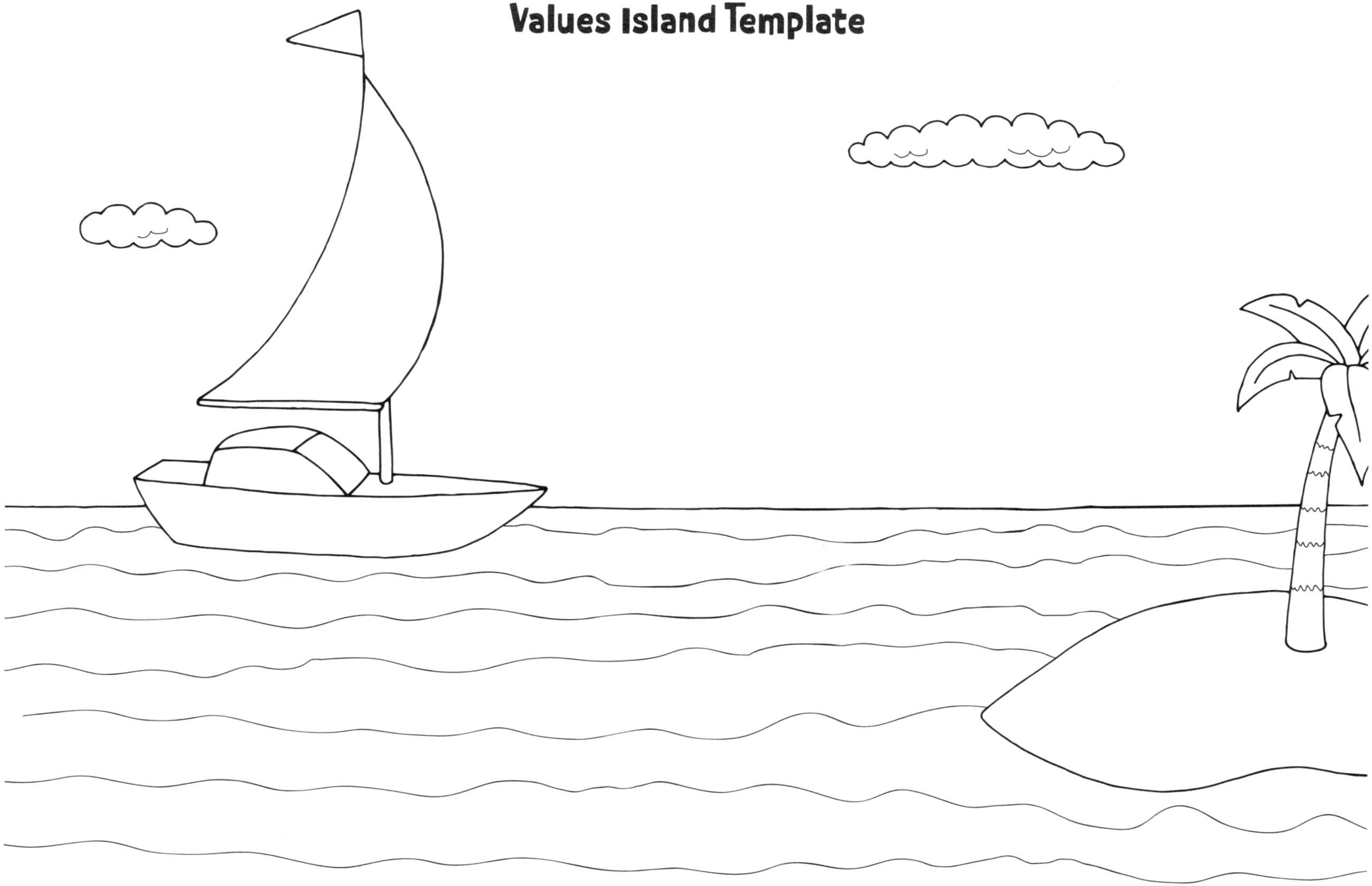

VPS: Values Positioning System

Therapeutic Rationale

This activity is designed as a follow-up to *Values Island*. While the previous activity is about identifying medium- and long-term committed actions, this one translates those values into moment-to-moment choices. In other words, it asks, "What are kids doing *today* to move them toward their values?" Just like a GPS helps us know where we are, remember where we want to go, and make adjustments when we get off track, a "values positioning system" helps kids pause and make choices that move them closer to what matters to them, even when things feel hard.

Goals

- Increase awareness of values-based actions in daily life
- Facilitate meaningful values-based actions

Materials

- None

Instructions

1. Begin by explaining that while big, dramatic actions can feel good, it's often the small, everyday choices we make that move us closer to a values-based life. These daily actions add up and guide the direction of our values.
2. Share with your client that just like a GPS guides us when we're driving, we also have a VPS—a values positioning system. The VPS helps us remember what matters most and reminds us which direction we want to move in to live a values-based life, especially when we're unsure or are tempted to take a different path.
3. Work with your client to identify what kinds of daily questions their VPS can help them answer—for example, "What choice moves me closer to my values right now?" and "What kind of person do I want to be in this situation?" Discuss how remembering their values can help guide difficult choices, like whether to do homework, go to sports practice, stick to their budget, and so on.
4. To close the activity, brainstorm strategies your client can use to help them stay committed to their values, even when they do not feel like it. This might include reminders, routines, visual cues, or affirmations.

Staying on the Path

Therapeutic Rationale

Many kids, particularly those who are neurodivergent, struggle to understand that "not right now" does not mean "never." This can make waiting, delaying gratification, and resisting impulses very difficult. An impulse is essentially a feeling of incredible thirst—but instead of water, it's a craving for a quick hit of dopamine. It's seeing a giant red button that says "Do Not Push" and immediately knowing that the only thing that they want in this world is to push that button. But the problem with chasing impulses is that it often gets in the way of fulfilling bigger, more meaningful goals. This exercise is designed to help kids stay on the path toward values-based committed action, even when their impulses are strong.

Goals

- Foster awareness of values and goals when faced with impulses
- Build strategies to resist impulses that could cause clients to "stray from the path"

Materials

- *Winding Path* template
- Writing utensil
- Crayons, markers, or colored pencils

Instructions

1. Ask your client if they've ever had an impulse that was hard to resist. You can share a funny story of your own if you'd like. For example, Matt often shares that when he sees a fire alarm, there is nothing more he wants to do than pull it!
2. Ask them what made them want to follow that impulse or what helped them resist it. Process the outcomes with them:
   a. How did it turn out (immediately and in long term) when they gave in to the impulse?
   b. How did it turn out (immediately and in the long term) when they resisted the impulse?
   c. Did giving in to the impulse move them closer to or farther away from their ultimate goal?

   Kiddos often struggle to see how impulses affect long-term goals or the privileges their caregivers give them. It can be beneficial to explicitly connect these dots for them.
3. Commiserate with your client: Sometimes, the world is full of "shiny things" pulling us off the path toward our goals. It can feel almost impossible to resist! Explain that you want to help them figure out strategies to stay on the path. Just like hiking requires attention and planning to stay on the right track, resisting impulses takes practice and the right tools to help them keep moving toward what matters most.
4. Introduce the *Winding Path* template, and ask your client about a recent time they got into trouble due to impulsive behavior. Help them identify what they did, which impulse

they were following, and which goal it prevented them from achieving. For example, if they got into trouble for fighting at school and they want to earn privileges to babysit their younger siblings for extra money, you could ask, "How did the fight help or hurt your parents' willingness to trust you with your siblings?"

5. Ask your client to choose one goal they want to work toward. This could be earning a better grade, getting a later bedtime, or improving at a sport—anything really, as long as it is meaningful to them. On the template, have them write their goal in the finish line.
6. Ask what impulses have gotten in the way of achieving this goal. Encourage them to think deeply and give real-world examples. Have them fill in these impulses along the winding path.
7. Next, brainstorm with your client: "How can we help you remember to stay on this path and not get lost in the woods?" Strategies may include remembering their values, using coping skills to regulate, or remembering that "not right now" does not mean "never." Have them write these strategies in the hiking bag at the start of the path.
8. Invite your client to share the completed template with their caregiver, explaining what they have learned and how they plan to use these ideas to prevent them from getting lost in the woods.

Winding Path Template

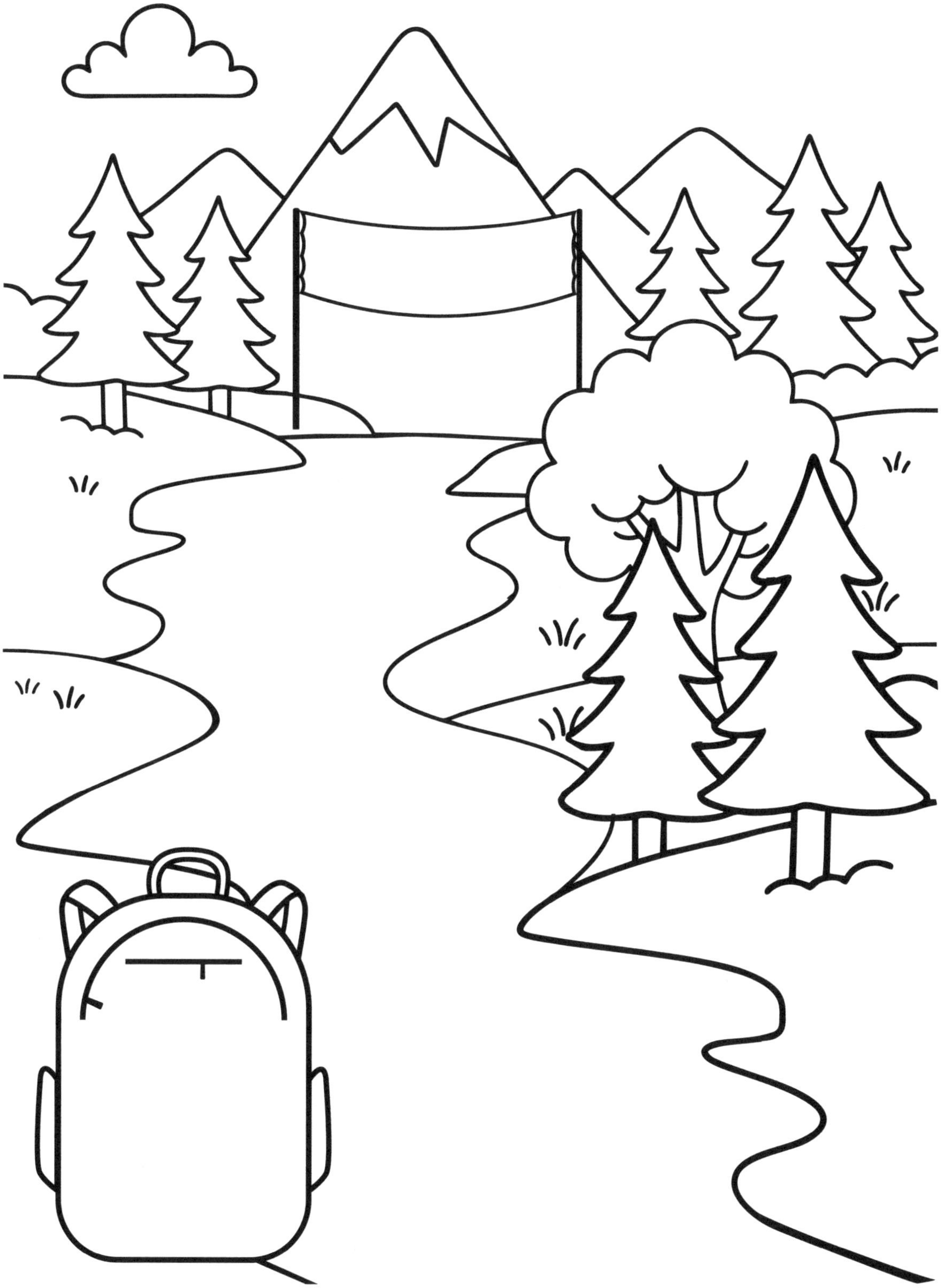

You've Got Mail

Therapeutic Rationale

While values act as a compass that guides us, kids often can forget to use their values—or forget which direction to move in. This activity helps kids remember their values, both in session and over time, in a creative, concrete, and meaningful way. By writing postcards to their future selves, kids create tangible reminders of what truly matters to them. When delivered later—either unexpectedly or at a predetermined time—these letters encourage kids to pause, reflect, and reorient toward their values.

Goals

- Create meaningful messages as a reminder to move toward values
- Reinforce values over time

Materials

- Blank postcards
- Writing utensil
- Stamps

Instructions

1. Introduce the idea that while values guide us, sometimes we need a little reminder or encouragement to stay on track. Ask the client to reflect on a day they felt stuck or unsure of how to move forward. What would they like to have heard on that day? It is those days we hope these cards can help.
2. Encourage the client to fill out a few postcards with kind, encouraging, and values-focused messages. They can be short or longer messages, as long as they're meaningful to the client. These can include positive affirmations, gentle reminders of past successes, or tips for coping with difficult situations. The client can also decorate the cards if they wish.
3. With the caregiver's permission, mail the postcards to the client at random times throughout the therapeutic relationship. If mailing isn't possible, hold onto the cards and ask the client to choose one at random during or after particularly challenging times.

What Lights You Up?

Therapeutic Rationale

Values are like electricity that powers the light inside of us—they help give us drive, motivation, and meaning. Just like every light needs a power source, we need daily practices, routines, and choices that help us stay connected to what matters most. This activity helps kids name both their core values and the actions or habits that help them recharge, allowing their light to keep shining bright even when life gets hard.

Goals

- Reflect on what energizes and motivates the client
- Identify actions or habits that support values-driven behavior

Materials

- *What Lights You Up?* template
- Writing utensil
- Crayons, markers, or colored pencils (optional)

Instructions

1. Introduce the activity: "Imagine you are powered by a light inside you. That light represents who you are at your core—your spark. When you do things that are consistent with your values, your light shines brighter. But when you feel stuck, tired, or take actions that don't move you toward your values, your light can get dim and need to be recharged. Today we are going to figure out not only what lights you up, but also what helps you recharge so your light can shine bright again!"
2. Ask the client to list the values that feel most important to them in the light bulb on the *What Lights You Up?* template. These are things that help the light shine bright.
3. For each value, ask what helps them engage in actions that align with that value. This could be a person who supports them, an activity they enjoy, a routine or habit, or a coping skill. Have them write these on the battery portion of the template. These are the actions that recharge their light so it can shine.
4. Give the client an opportunity to decorate or add to the template if they want to.

What Lights You Up? Template

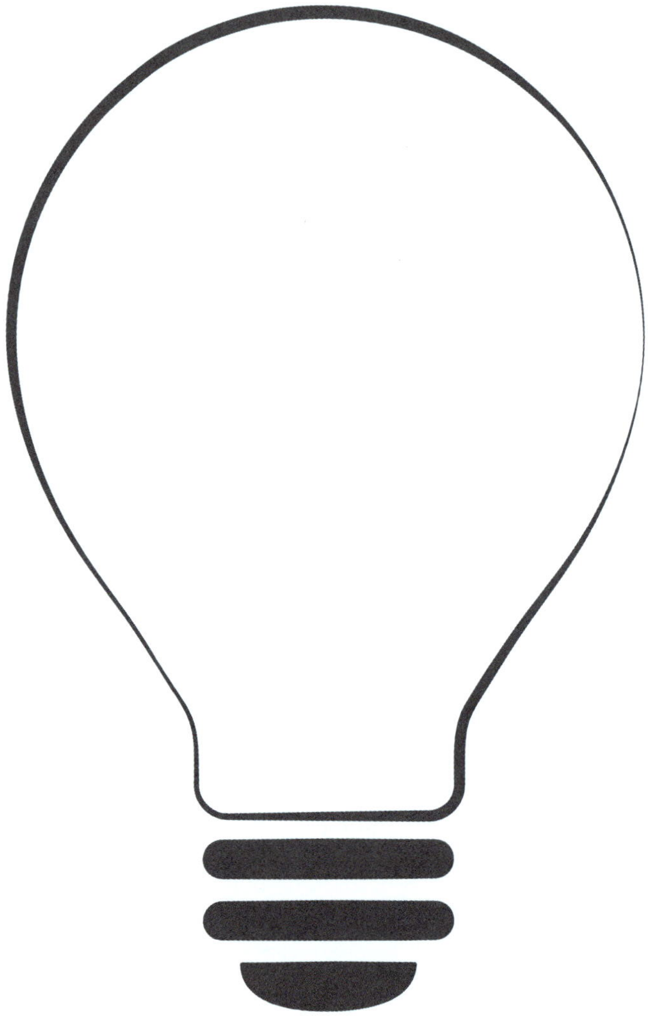

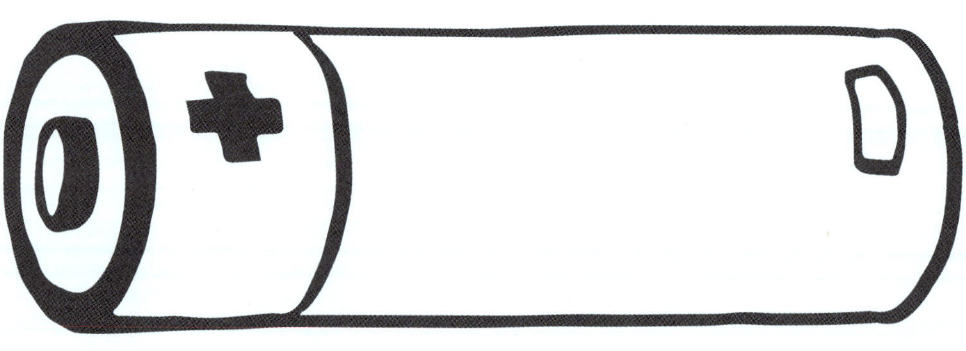

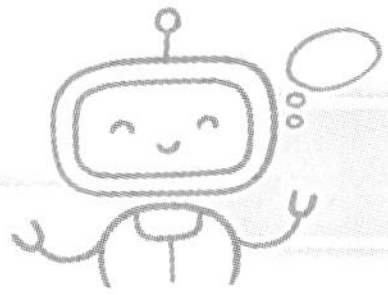

Noticing Impulses

Therapeutic Rationale

In the previous *Staying on the Path* activity, we talked about the difference between giving in to impulses and delaying gratification. While some impulses can prevent us from reaching our goals, others can actually be helpful! This can include the impulse to offer kind words to a friend, to help clear the table after a meal, or include someone who is being left out. This activity helps kids notice and nurture the helpful impulses while moving away from hurtful impulses.

Goals

- Increase awareness of helpful versus unhelpful impulses
- Encourage helpful impulsive behaviors while decreasing unhelpful ones

Materials

- *Noticing Impulses* worksheet
- Writing utensil

Instructions

1. Ask the client if they think all impulses are bad or whether some are useful. Explain that, as with most things, impulses can sometimes help us, sometimes get us into trouble, or sometimes do a little of both.
2. Use the *Noticing Impulses* worksheet to help the client brainstorm examples from their own life:
   a. Times when an impulse led to something positive (e.g., saying something kind)
   b. Times when an impulse caused problems (e.g., grabbing something without asking)
3. Go through each entry together, asking what made that action helpful or hurtful. Often, helpfulness can be measured by the impact it had on them or others.
   a. "What did you notice about the impulses that helped?"
   b. "What did you notice about the impulses that caused problems?"
   c. "How did you feel when you acted on each impulse?"
   d. "What are some early warning signs that an impulse is coming, and how can you tell whether it's likely to help or cause problems?"
4. Brainstorm strategies to recognize these warning signs. How will they know that it is time to stop, take a breath, and consider their next move? Strategies might include counting to 10, asking for help, or thinking about the outcomes before acting.
5. Give the client a clean copy of the worksheet to take home. Have them complete it with their caregiver each day (or as often as possible) and bring it to the next session. Review their entries together, celebrate their wins, and continue refining strategies for increasing helpful impulses while decreasing unhelpful ones.

Noticing Impulses Worksheet

Use this worksheet to keep track of your impulses, notice how they affect you and others, and decide whether they are more helpful or more harmful.

Impulse	How Was It Helpful?	How Was It Unhelpful?	Was It More Helpful or More Unhelpful?

Your Superpowers

Therapeutic Rationale

One of the most appealing elements of ACT is its holistic focus. It is about helping people live meaningful lives—not just the absence of illness. Part of that involves finding joy in life and in ourselves. Life is this strange, absurd, and wonderful thing that we all are privileged enough to experience, but we often get so caught up in our worries or frustrations that we forget a critical element of wellness: celebrating the qualities that make us uniquely *us*. Each of us is a remarkable mix of quirks, strengths, and traits, so instead of feeling self-conscious about it, why not revel in it? This activity helps kids recognize what makes them special and reframe self-conscious thoughts into personal "superpowers."

Goals

- Reframe negative self-talk into positive, empowering statements
- Instill greater self-confidence and courage in identity

Materials

- *Your Superpowers* worksheet
- Writing utensil

Instructions

1. Ask your client about their favorite superhero. What are the character's superpowers? What do they like about the character? What traits do they find silly or amusing? What traits do they feel like they share with the character?
2. Ask if everyone knows the superhero's secret identity. Of course not! Explain that, just like a superhero, people don't always see your client's full self. Sometimes, others make assumptions based on what they can see, which can make your client feel judged.
3. Using the *Your Superpowers* worksheet, work with your client to identify traits or interests they feel self-conscious about. Maybe it's a hobby that isn't "cool" or an activity they enjoy that they're "too old for." Unfortunately, kids can be unkind and judgmental, so you'll likely have plenty of examples to work with.
4. For each entry, help them notice any unhelpful self-talk, particularly hidden assumptions: "If I do/am this, then that means ________ about me." Often, this reveals an implicit belief that others won't like them or that they might end up alone (or be unworthy of love).
5. Help them "superpower-ify" this negative self-talk by reframing it into affirming statements. For example, "I'm a nerd if I like fantasy games" can become "I have such a vivid imagination!"
6. Discuss how these superpowers can help them feel great about themselves, no matter what anyone else thinks. Nobody knows that Superman is Clark Kent, but *he* knows. Your client knows who they are, and if they lean into it, they will ultimately feel better about themselves.

Your Superpowers Worksheet

Use this worksheet to identify qualities about yourself that make you feel self-conscious, notice any mean or negative thoughts you tell yourself about these qualities, and turn them into your own personal superpowers.

Quality, Attribute, or Interest	**Unhelpful Self-Talk**	**Superpower-ify it!** (Turn it into more helpful self-talk)

Values Poster

Therapeutic Rationale

When we take the time to see our values written out, as opposed to only talking about them, they can feel more real, more integrated, and more accessible in our daily lives. Creating a personalized values poster gives kids a chance to reflect on what matters most and express those values creatively. This process supports motivation from within while also providing external reminders of what matters most. By choosing to display the poster in a meaningful space, such as their room, they can intentionally connect to their values in everyday moments.

Goals

- Reflect on and consolidate values in a mindful, creative way
- Increase motivation and connection with values

Materials

- Poster board
- Crayons, markers, or colored pencils
- Craft items (e.g., photos, stickers, glitter, glue) (optional)

Instructions

1. Introduce the activity: "We've spent a lot of time talking about what matters to you and what guides you forward—your values. Today we're going to create a poster with your values on them so you can see them in front of you!"
2. Ask the client to think about what values they want to include on their poster. It might be helpful to look back on previous values activities if needed.
3. Design the poster, allowing the client to fill it in and decorate it however they would like. If they need help writing out values, you can assist, but it's important that they have a chance to personalize the design.
4. Encourage the client to work slowly and thoughtfully, making sure they know that there is no wrong way to create or decorate the poster.
5. Once the poster is complete, allow the client to take it home. Encourage them to hang it up somewhere where they will see it daily. Suggest that they spend a few moments each day looking at it and reflecting on how they can act on their values.
6. **Optional:** The client can create a shared values poster together with their family or household. This can help everyone reflect together on what is most important to them as a whole and support each other by living those values.

Gut Check Journal

Therapeutic Rationale

We all have gut feelings—sometimes we just *know* something without being able to verbalize why. Learning to listen to these feelings, discern what they might be signaling, and know when to trust them is a valuable skill. In this activity, kids will track their gut feelings, notice how their body responds in different situations, and reflect on what these signals might be telling them about their choices. This helps kids connect their instincts to their values, emotions, and actions, supporting decision-making that aligns with what matters most.

Goals

- Practice noticing and listening to gut feelings
- Develop awareness of the connection between body sensations, emotions, and actions

Materials

- *Gut Check* worksheet
- Writing utensil
- Feelings wheel (optional)

Instructions

1. Talk with your client about what having a "gut feeling" means to them. How do they know when it's their gut talking? Do they find it easy or difficult to listen to their gut? What makes it easier or difficult?
2. Explain that learning to listen to and trust their gut takes practice. To help, they'll keep a weekly log using the *Gut Check* worksheet. For each entry, they should write the following:
    a. What happened (e.g., the situation that triggered their gut feeling)
    b. How their body felt during and after the event (e.g., tense, butterflies, energy)
    c. What emotions they experienced (e.g., happiness, anxiety)
    d. What message they think their body was trying to send (e.g., trying warn them, encourage them)
3. Some clients benefit from using a feelings wheel as they complete the worksheet.
4. Have the client bring the log to session each week. Process their entries together by reviewing any noteworthy events, emotional insights, or gut messages they may have missed. Discuss how these feelings or gut reactions might relate to their values or influence their actions. For example, did they feel more aligned or disconnected from their values when they listened to their gut?

Gut Check Worksheet

Use this worksheet to track specific events, situations, or moments throughout the week when you had a strong gut feeling about something. Describe how your body felt during and after that event, what emotions popped up, and what you think your body might have been trying to tell you.

Date	What Happened?	How Did Your Body Feel During and After?	What Emotions Did You Experience?	What Message Was Your Body Trying to Send?

Values Reflection

Therapeutic Rationale

This activity supports children in the ongoing practice of mindful values-based living. It encourages them to slow down and check in with where they are, which allows them build self-awareness and make more intentional, values-based choices. It also highlights that it's okay to make small course corrections along the way rather than expecting to be perfect all the time.

Goals

- Promote mindful self-awareness in relation to values
- Strengthen the ability to make values-based decisions in different situations

Materials

- Blank paper
- Writing utensil

Instructions

1. Ask the client to take a deep breath and then reflect or write their responses to the following questions:
    a. "What value or personal quality has felt most important to you lately?" (*Examples might include kindness, honesty, growth, creativity, connection, fun, or courage.*)
    b. "In the past few days, what is one thing you did that moved you *toward* this value?" (*What action, decision, or moment felt "right" or meaningful?*)
    c. "Was there a moment when you moved *away* from this value, maybe because you were tired, stressed, scared, or distracted?" (*No need to judge, just notice.*)
    d. "What thoughts or feelings showed up when you tried to live your values?" (*Did anything get in the way?*)
    e. "How do you feel when you're acting in line with what matters to you?" (*And how does it feel when you're not?*)
    f. "What's one small thing you can do today that moves you closer to your values?" (*Try this, even if it's only one step closer.*)
2. Encourage clients to repeat this reflection at home as needed. Some may benefit from practicing it daily or several times per week, while others may need it less frequently. However, a good starting point is a few times a week and gradually tapering down as it becomes part of their routine. It can also be helpful to do the reflection briefly at the start or end of a session.

Moments of Meaning

Therapeutic Rationale

This activity encourages kids to become more mindful of how often they already act in alignment with their values—even in small, everyday moments. By tracking these moments, kids learn to notice, savor, and reinforce behaviors that reflect what truly matters to them. This builds self-efficacy, emotional clarity, and a stronger sense of purpose.

Goals

- Increase awareness of values-consistent actions
- Promote mindfulness in daily routines
- Strengthen the link between actions and internal values

Materials

- *Moments of Meaning* worksheet
- Writing utensil

Instructions

1. Introduce the activity: "Today we're going to start paying attention to the small and big things you do throughout the day that feel meaningful or important to you—the moments when you think, 'This matters.'"
2. Decide whether to track these moments daily or weekly. Choose a frequency that is both developmentally appropriate and sustainable for the client.
3. At the end of each day (or week, depending on your tracking period), invite the client to pause and reflect on these guiding questions:
    a. "Did I do anything today that reflected who I want to be or what I care about?"
    b. "Was there a moment when I felt [*proud, connected, kind, strong, helpful, honest, etc.*]?" Adjust the list of values to reflect those they have previously identified.
4. Instruct the client to record each moment on the *Moments of Meaning* worksheet. They should make sure to note the following:
    a. What action they took
    b. The value this moment reflected (e.g., honesty, family, kindness, fun)
    c. How they felt before, during, and after the moment
    d. Why the moment felt meaningful to them
5. At the next session, review the moments together. Look for themes, surprises, and signs of growth.

Moments of Meaning Worksheet

Each day (or week), write down moments that felt important or meaningful to you.

What Action Did You Take?	What Value Did This Reflect?	How Did You Feel Before, During, and After?	Why Did It Feel Meaningful?

Values Kite

Therapeutic Rationale

Mindfulness isn't just about calming down or sitting still—it's about tuning in. This activity helps kids notice what it feels like to hold onto their values while also letting go of the need to control everything around them. Flying a kite provides a concrete, sensory-rich metaphor for this: They can hold the string, but they can't control the wind. In the same way, they can connect to their values even when the world feels unpredictable.

Goals

- Promote values awareness through an embodied outdoor experience
- Connect the concept of "holding on" to values with "letting go" of control
- Build flexibility and resilience when moving toward what matters

Materials

- Simple kite (purchased or homemade)
- Permanent marker
- Safe space outside to fly a kite

Instructions

1. Introduce the activity: "Today we're going to do something a little different. We're going to fly a kite, but not just any kite. This kite represents your values—the things that matter most to you. As you fly it, you'll get to feel what it's like to hold on to those values while letting them rise and shift in the wind."
2. Invite the client to write three to five values on the kite using a permanent marker. You may revisit previous values activities or use the *Values Foundation* worksheet (see page 198) to help them choose.
3. Now it's time to fly the kite! Go outside together (or assign this as a take-home activity). As the client flies the kite, invite them to notice:
   a. The feeling of the string in their hand
   b. How the wind moves the kite in unexpected ways
   c. How they stay connected even when the kite feels far away
   d. What it's like to watch their values soaring
4. Afterward, reflect on how the experience relates to their everyday life—how they can stay connected to their values even when they cannot control what is happening around them.

SECTION 6

Committed Action

In ACT, committed action is about taking meaningful steps toward the things that matter to us—even when, or perhaps especially when, it feels hard. It is not about being perfect, fearless, or always getting it right. Instead, it's about choosing to move in the direction of our values, one step at a time, with flexibility, courage, and care.

This kind of action takes intention and patience. It invites us to continue showing up for ourselves again and again, even when our motivation is low or the path forward is unclear. For kids, this might look like raising their hand in class even when they feel nervous (because learning is important to them), persevering at a sport or instrument even when they're frustrated (because trying their best matters), including a peer who has been left out even if it feels awkward (because kindness matters), or apologizing after making a mistake even when it feels hard (because it's important to be accountable).

You might find it helpful to explain committed action as the bridge between values and behavior. Whereas acceptance, mindfulness, and defusion help kids create the space to notice what is happening inside them, committed action gives them a way forward—a chance to act if you will!

Values vs. Goals

Therapeutic Rationale

Values are the deep, guiding principles that give life direction and meaning, such as kindness, creativity, and honesty. Goals, however, are the specific and actionable steps we take that move us closer to living by those values. Goals can, and indeed should, be achieved over time, while values are ongoing and always available to return to. This activity helps kids differentiate between values and goals, but more than that, learn how to use their values to develop goals that keep them moving in a meaningful direction.

Goals

- Clarify the difference between values (the direction we move in) and goals (the destination)
- Create goals that align with personal values

Materials

- *Values vs. Goals* worksheet
- Writing utensil

Instructions

1. Introduce the activity: "Values are like a compass—they help us decide what direction we want to go in life. Goals, on the other hand, are like checkpoints or destinations on a map. We use our values to guide us toward our goals, and if we keep moving, we are able to reach our goals over time."
2. Ask clients about goals they have achieved, or share some of your own. For example:
   a. **Value:** Being a lifelong learner ⇒ **Goal:** Getting an advanced degree
   b. **Value:** Being a supportive sibling ⇒ **Goal:** Going to their soccer games and cheering them on
3. Provide your client with the *Value vs. Goals* worksheet and have them write their values (which they should have identified in previous activities) in the left-hand column. Then ask them to create one or more goals that reflects that value in the right-hand column.
4. There is no right or wrong number of goals, but keep in mind that some goals should be ones you can work on in sessions with them. Goals like "get an A on this test" are wonderful and certainly have a place, but they are more challenging to work on in session.
5. Over the next week, ask them to work on one or more of their goals, using their values as a guide. Encourage small, achievable steps.
6. Follow up! At the start of the next session, check in on their progress. Which goals did they work on this week? Which values helped them toward those goals?

Values vs. Goals Worksheet

Write down your values in the left column. For each value, create a goal in the right column that reflects that value.

Your Value	Your Goal

Goal Mapping

Therapeutic Rationale

Values guide us toward meaningful growth, while goals help us take action toward that growth. However, goals can also lend themselves to all-or-nothing thinking. Kids may share big goals, like "My goal is to climb Mount Everest!" and feel despondent when they have not reached the summit by the next session. This activity is designed to remind them that goals are tools to serve a meaningful life, not vice versa. That is, goals exist solely to help us move toward that which is most important to us. They act as signposts that help us reflect on our direction and progress, ensuring that we are still moving in the direction that it is most meaningful for us to go in.

Goals

- Expand psychological flexibility surrounding goals
- Set short-, medium-, and long-term goals to facilitate committed action

Materials

- *Goal Mapping* worksheet
- Blank paper
- Writing utensil

Instructions

1. Ask your client to share some goals they have that are reflective of their values. These can range from big to small—all goals are welcome! Have them write down these goals on a blank piece of paper and share why they selected these particular goals.
2. Explain that goals are like road signs that help us see where we're going in life. These road signs let us know the direction we're moving in and help us decide if we want to continue in that direction. If not, we can always use our *value positioning system* (VPS)—like a GPS—to choose a new direction.
3. Ask your client to break down their goals into short-term, medium-term, and long-term categories. Encourage your client to think about what needs to happen for each goal, then categorize each one accordingly on the *Goal Mapping* worksheet.
    a. **Short-term goals** are things that can be achieved in the immediate future (e.g., "I want to read two books this month").
    b. **Medium-term goals** are achievable in a few months (e.g., "I want to improve my soccer skills by the end of the semester").
    c. **Long-term goals** take longer to achieve and are more ambitious (e.g., "I want to make the varsity soccer team next year").
4. Discuss how long-term and medium-term goals often require smaller, shorter-term goals to achieve them. For example, if the long-term goal is to climb Mount Everest, a

short-term goal may be to create a training plan. Brainstorm what shorter-term steps they can take to achieve their medium- and long-term goals.

5. Encourage your client to reflect on the actions they are taking each day. Are those actions moving them closer to or further away from their goals? For instance, if a client's goal is to make the basketball team, but they haven't been practicing at all, discuss how this habit may be interfering with their goal.
6. Remind your client that goals do not have to be permanent. They should reflect on their goals at least two or three times per year to determine whether they are still moving in the direction that aligns with their values.

Goal Mapping Worksheet

Write down your goals for the next few weeks, months, and the future. Then think about the steps you need to take to reach those goals.

Long-Term Goals (6+ months)	**Medium-Term Goals (3–6 months)**	**Short-Term Goals (1–3 months)**

What's in Your Backpack? Part 2

Therapeutic Rationale

In part 1 of this activity (see page 70), we explored how managing trauma can be like wearing an overloaded backpack. It weighs you down, is always with you, and feels like there is no better way to manage it. In this follow-up activity, we continue using this metaphor to address the process of committed action, especially when it comes to committing to treatment. Some kids might feel ambivalent about (or even find comfort in) their struggles because that's what's familiar to them. They may commit to treatment on a surface level while demonstrating an ongoing reluctance to take steps to actually feel better. This activity is designed to help work through that resistance.

Goals

- Reduce ambivalence about engaging in therapy
- Explore fears about engaging in treatment

Materials

- Backpack
- Variety of books

Instructions

1. Before starting this activity, complete part 1 of *What's in Your Backpack?* to ensure your client has already explored what it's like to carry their emotional "load."
2. Tell your client that it seems like they have been hesitant to take books out of their backpack, and you want to explore why that might be. Ask them directly whether they agree with your inference. Have they been hesitant to remove the books from the backpack (i.e., engage in therapy)?
3. Share that sometimes it feels safer and more comfortable to leave the books where they are. It can be scary to move them because the client can't predict what will happen when they do. What if they try and feel worse? What if they fail? Worse yet, what if they *succeed?* Sometimes, the idea that we might actually feel better is the scariest thing of all.
4. Gently explore the idea that depression, anxiety, and other struggles can feel comfortable because they are familiar. What scares your client about trying to make the change? What scares them about failing? What scares them about succeeding?
5. Discuss how taking committed action in therapy doesn't mean forcing change all at once. It's about committing to *try* to feel better. Ask your client what has to occur for them to be willing to do that. Brainstorm ideas, if necessary.
6. If they're willing, have them remove some books from the backpack and wear it again, but with a lighter load. Ask how it feels to carry a lighter backpack.

7. Conclude by discussing the idea of hope. Explain that most people think hope is the belief that tomorrow *will* be better, but that's incorrect. Hope is the belief that tomorrow *can* be better. It's time to hope.

Goal Getting

Therapeutic Rationale

Many kids struggle with the process of achieving their goals. While they can identify their goals and understand the values behind them, it can be much more challenging to take actionable steps toward those goals. This activity helps kids break down larger goals into smaller checkpoints—or "mini" goals—to help them track their progress toward their larger goals. It also reminds them that goal getting isn't always a straight line and that setbacks are a part of the journey.

Goals

- Create a plan to make progress toward goals
- Build checkpoints to recognize and celebrate progress
- Understand that goal achievement is not always a linear process

Materials

- *Goal Getting* template
- Writing utensil

Instructions

1. Introduce the activity: "Have you ever seen a soccer field? On each side of the field are two nets, and the goal is to kick the ball into the net. But how do you actually get the ball across the field? That's what we are going to explore today. We're going to figure out the steps to get your ball (i.e., your goal) across the field and strategize what to do if the other team steals the ball."
2. Ask your client to write one or more of their goals by the soccer net on the *Goal Getting* template. This is their ultimate goal—the "big picture" they're aiming for.
3. Help them break down this goal into achievable steps. For example, if their goal is to make more friends, some steps might include joining a new club or hobby, introducing themselves to someone new, finding a shared interest, or asking someone to hang out. Have them write these steps in the lines on the field.
4. Discuss how in soccer, when the other team steals the ball, the players have to run backward down the field. But that doesn't mean the game is lost! Similarly, when the client has a setback in reaching their goals, it doesn't negate how far they have come. It just means they may need to try a new route with an additional checkpoint or two.
5. Note that some goals may have more checkpoints than others, and that is okay! For example, the long-term goal of becoming an astronaut is going to have more checkpoints than a short-term goal of diving in the deep end of the pool by the end of summer. That is to be expected.
6. Close the activity by reinforcing the idea that every little step counts, even when they face a setback. The goal is to stay flexible and keep moving toward what matters most to them.

Goal Getting Template

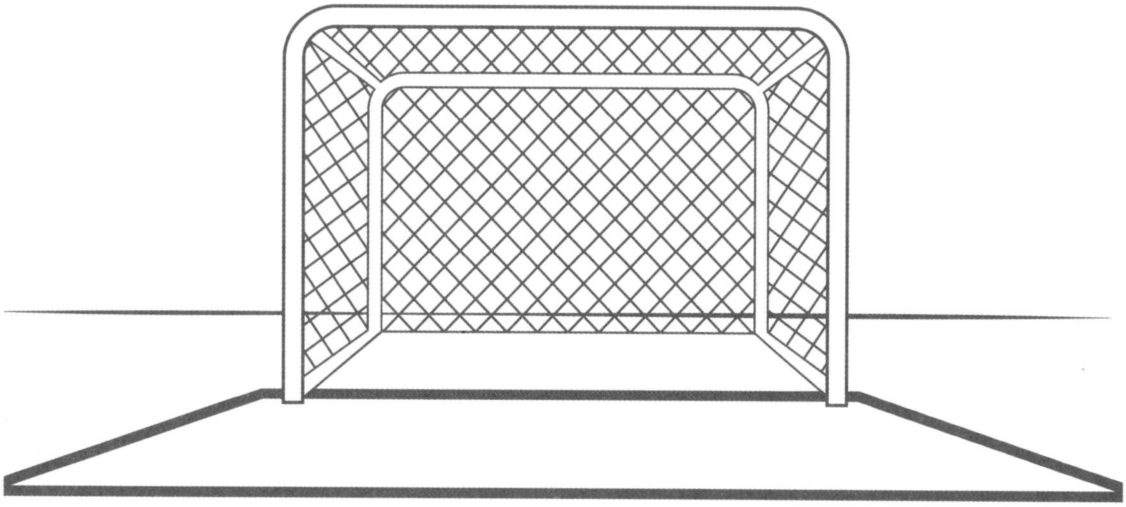

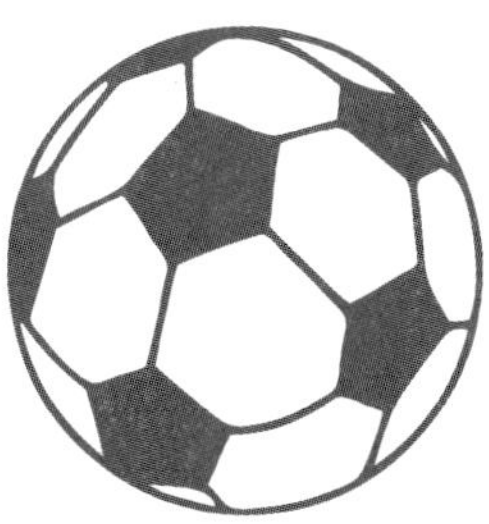

Acting as If

Therapeutic Rationale

There is a very amusing genre of internet videos where people confidently "act as if" they belong in a particular place or situation—and somehow they're accepted in that role! For example, one video shows a person walking backstage at a concert wearing a safety vest and carrying a clipboard, as if they're part of the crew to meet their favorite band. Another shows someone strolling into the Super Bowl without any tickets! While we certainly don't condone breaking any laws, we do believe the underlying lesson is important: Sometimes, it really is as simple as "fake it 'til you make it." That's what this activity helps kids do.

Goals

- Build self-confidence
- Take meaningful action that reflects all six elements of the hexaflex

Materials

- Computer with speakers

Instructions

1. Begin by showing your client videos of people who are "acting as if"—confidently stepping into situations where they don't seem to belong but are accepted because of their self-confidence. Remember to screen the videos beforehand to make sure you're not encouraging your client to do anything illegal or inappropriate!
2. Ask your client what allows the people in the videos to act this way. Point out that, at its core, it's about confidence—confidence that it is okay to be who they are, be where they are, and do what they are doing.
3. Discuss what they believe gets in the way of their ability to feel that type of confidence. Does anxiety get the better of them? Do they catastrophize and assume that things will go wrong before they even try?
4. Introduce the idea of "acting as if" they already have that confidence. What would it be like if they pretended for a moment that their anxiety, depression, or fear was not in control of their life? What might that look like? What might they be able to accomplish?
5. It's normal for clients to be skeptical. If that happens, explain that "acting as if" does not erase those uncomfortable feelings, but a funny thing happens when they "act as if" for long enough: It starts to feel real. The only real difference between fake confidence and real confidence is action.
6. Brainstorm some ways your client could begin to "act as if" in small, manageable ways. Could they try this at school or in an extracurricular activity?

7. Assign a small "acting as if" task for homework. Make sure it's a step they feel comfortable with but also stretches them a little. In the next session, review how it went. Encourage your client to keep practicing, as this is an activity that becomes more helpful the more they return to it.

Miracle Question

Therapeutic Rationale

Composer Igor Stravinsky once said, "Good composers borrow, great composers steal." While we wouldn't go so far as to steal, we do embrace the idea of borrowing helpful concepts from other therapeutic traditions. Once such concept is the *Miracle Question*, which comes to us from solution-focused therapy. This exercise invites kids to imagine that a miracle occurred overnight, solving all of their problems. When they wake up the next day, what would they notice first? How would they know things were different? Here, we take the miracle question and add an ACT twist to it.

Goals

- Make change appear less daunting and more achievable
- Foster the belief in the possibility of meaningful change
- Engage in committed action toward desired change

Materials

- None

Instructions

1. Introduce the miracle question: "Imagine that when you go to sleep tonight, a miracle happens. Overnight, everything in your life is suddenly 'fixed.' When you wake up tomorrow, what would you notice? What would be different?"
2. Give your client a few moments to consider their response. Many kids will mention grand ideas, like "I would be a billionaire" or "I would be invincible." While these are fun to think about, encourage them to stay within the realm of what is possible. Process their response, making sure to discuss what they would feel, think, and do in this situation.
3. Once they've shared, explain, "Unfortunately, a miracle is probably not going to happen tonight. While that's a bummer, it's also a reminder of something pretty cool: I'm willing to bet that we can figure out a plan to move you at least a little bit closer to that miracle outcome. Even if we can't accomplish it all in one night, I bet we can get you just 1 percent closer. What's one thing you can realistically do that will allow you to get even 1 percent closer to that goal?"
4. Brainstorm ideas with your client. After that first 1 percent, what does the next 1 percent look like? How about the 1 percent after that? Dare we dream big and consider what a 2 percent step might look like? Come up with an action plan and assign it as homework!
5. Remind your client that small steps add up over time. For example, 1 percent improvement per day can quickly add up to 5 percent, 10 percent, or even 50 percent. Goals often seem much harder to reach than they actually are, and taking small steps can lead to big change.

Locus of Control

Therapeutic Rationale

It's so easy for kids, and even for us as clinicians, to feel stuck or trapped by the things we cannot control. Shifting the focus to what *is* within our control can create momentum toward meaningful action. This is especially true for kids who struggle with the idea of "I can't" or who have difficulty starting. This activity encourages them to focus on the things they can control rather than getting overwhelmed by what's out of their control.

Goals

- Shift the focus from what is beyond one's control to what one can control
- Encourage taking the first steps toward a goal
- Overcome the "I can't" mindset

Materials

- *Locus of Control* worksheet
- Writing utensil

Instructions

1. Introduce the activity: "It can be really overwhelming when it feels like nothing is in our control. It's easy to get caught up in the things we can't control, and that can make it hard to take steps toward our goals."
2. Introduce the *Locus of Control* worksheet, pointing out that the page is mostly blank. That blank space represents the sea of things that are out of the client's control. The smaller circle in the middle represents the things they *can* control. Explain that even though the circle is smaller than the bigger area, the things inside it can have a huge impact on their life.
3. If the client struggles to grasp the idea, give them an example of the weather. Weather is inherently out of our control. We can't change it, but we can decide how to respond to it. We can notice it, plan for it, and adjust our actions based on it. Or we can decide to never leave the house if the weather isn't perfect.
4. Ask your client to list some things they can control and write them in the middle circle. If they have trouble coming up with ideas, ask them to think about what they chose to wear today, who they decide to play with at recess, who they decide to talk to, and so on.
5. Emphasize that by focusing on the things within their control, they can start taking meaningful steps toward their goals. It requires a constant and conscious choice to focus on what is within their control and move toward their values and goals.

Locus of Control Template

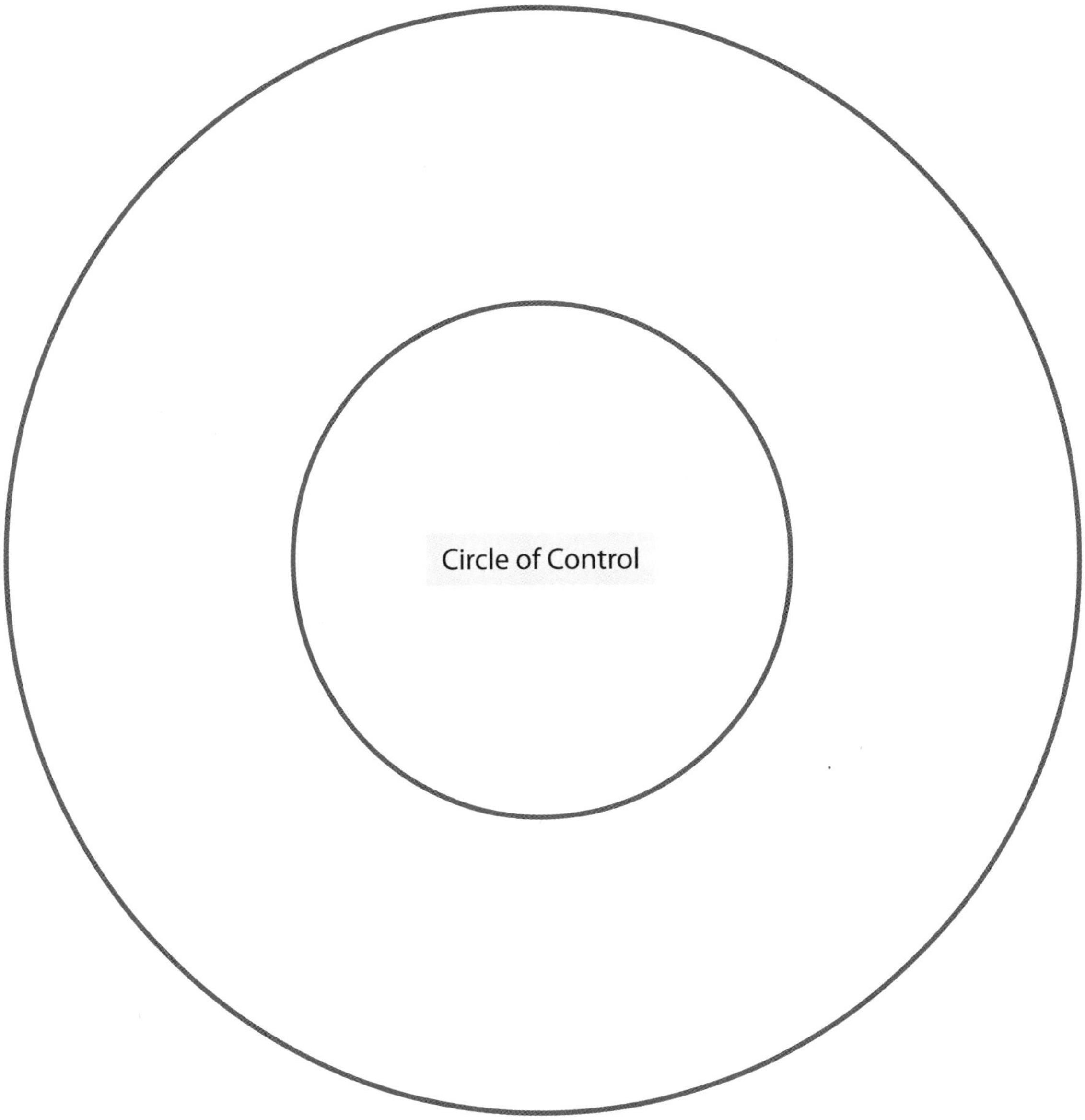

Three True Choices

Therapeutic Rationale

We have all experienced kids who seem to be maddeningly stuck in the precontemplation stage of change. These are the kids who, despite any reflection, affirmation, support, or challenging, seem to respond with some variation of "But it's haaaaarrrrrrddd!" We have exhaustive knowledge of this on a personal level—because we both do this exact thing as clients. We will complain, avoid, and sit in the comfort of misery. This exercise is designed to help clients like us. It is most effective when it is shared after a child has brought up a topic that has been discussed extensively in therapy, but they seem unwilling to work on it.

Goals

- Gain clarity about the motivations behind action (or inaction)
- Address avoidance behavior
- Facilitate movement toward a different stage of change

Materials

- None

Instructions

1. Explain that any time we're faced with an uncomfortable or difficult situation, there are really only three choices we can make. Allow them to guess what those choices may be.
2. Share with them that the three choices are: (1) complain, (2) work to accept it, or (3) work to change it.
3. Give your client a moment to consider whether there are any options outside of these three. They likely won't be able to think of one.
4. Explain that complaining is actually a wonderful first step because it helps us recognize what's not working or what we don't like. However, if we stay stuck on complaining without moving on to one of the other two choices, we lose the power to change the situation or our perspective.
5. Ask your client to think about a situation that they've been avoiding, resisting, or struggling with. Ideally, it should be something they've discussed in therapy before.
6. With that situation in mind, ask, "What has to happen for you to be ready to move to acceptance (choice 2) or change (choice 3)?"
7. Give them time to consider what you are saying, but if they're resistant to move forward, challenge them: "What is so comfortable about choice 1? What makes it worth giving up your power? What is scary about moving on to choice 2 or 3?"

8. Once they've reflected, ask your client what they want to try first: choice 2 or 3. Brainstorm strategies for doing so. If they are *really* stuck on choice 1, discuss what has to happen for them to feel ready to take action. Assign it as homework and then return to it in another session.

Playing Your Position

Therapeutic Rationale

Growing up involves figuring out who we are and what we want to be in life. Just like in soccer, kids can choose different "positions" in life, depending on the situation, to move them toward their values and goals. They can also ask for help or switch roles to make reaching those goals easier. While this activity uses the game of soccer as a metaphor, feel free to adapt it to whatever sport or activity is most relevant for your kiddo.

Goals

- Consider when to engage in different roles in life
- Engage in meaningful, committed action that aligns with desires, values, and goals

Materials

- *Soccer Field* worksheet
- Writing utensil

Instructions

1. Explain that in a game of soccer, different players fill different positions, each with specific responsibilities:
    a. **Strikers** are aggressive offensive players who focus on scoring.
    b. **Midfielders** play both offense and defense, moving around the field depending on the situation.
    c. **Defenders** work with the goalkeeper to prevent the other team from scoring.
    d. **Goalkeepers** are responsible for protecting the goal and stopping the ball.

    Consider other positions as well, such as referees, coaches, or even fans.

1. Ask your client if they have a favorite position in soccer and explore why they like it. What strengths or qualities do they associate with it?
2. Introduce the idea that life is like a soccer field, where we move toward our desired goal even if it seems far away sometimes. Have your client write down their goals, desires, and values in the goal area of the *Soccer Field* worksheet.
3. Now have them fill in the four positions on the field, considering which positions might help them move closer to their goals and values. For example:
    a. **Striker:** What actions can they take to pursue their goals?
    b. **Midfielder:** How can they stay flexible, shifting roles as needed?
    c. **Defense:** When facing setbacks, what can they do to protect their progress?
    d. **Keeper:** How can they keep the goals they've achieved safe?

4. Discuss whether they'll need to switch between positions depending on the situation. For example, they might need to shift from being a striker to a defender when obstacles arise. Emphasize what "plays" or committed actions they can take to move forward toward their goal. Feel free to expand the metaphor as appropriate, considering how different "positions" and "plays" in life help us achieve our goals.

Soccer Field Worksheet

Use this worksheet to map out your goals, values, and desires, as well as the roles (striker, midfielder, defender, goalkeeper) you can play to move toward them.

Keeper

How can you keep the goals you've achieved safe?

Midfielder

How can you stay flexible, shifting roles as needed?

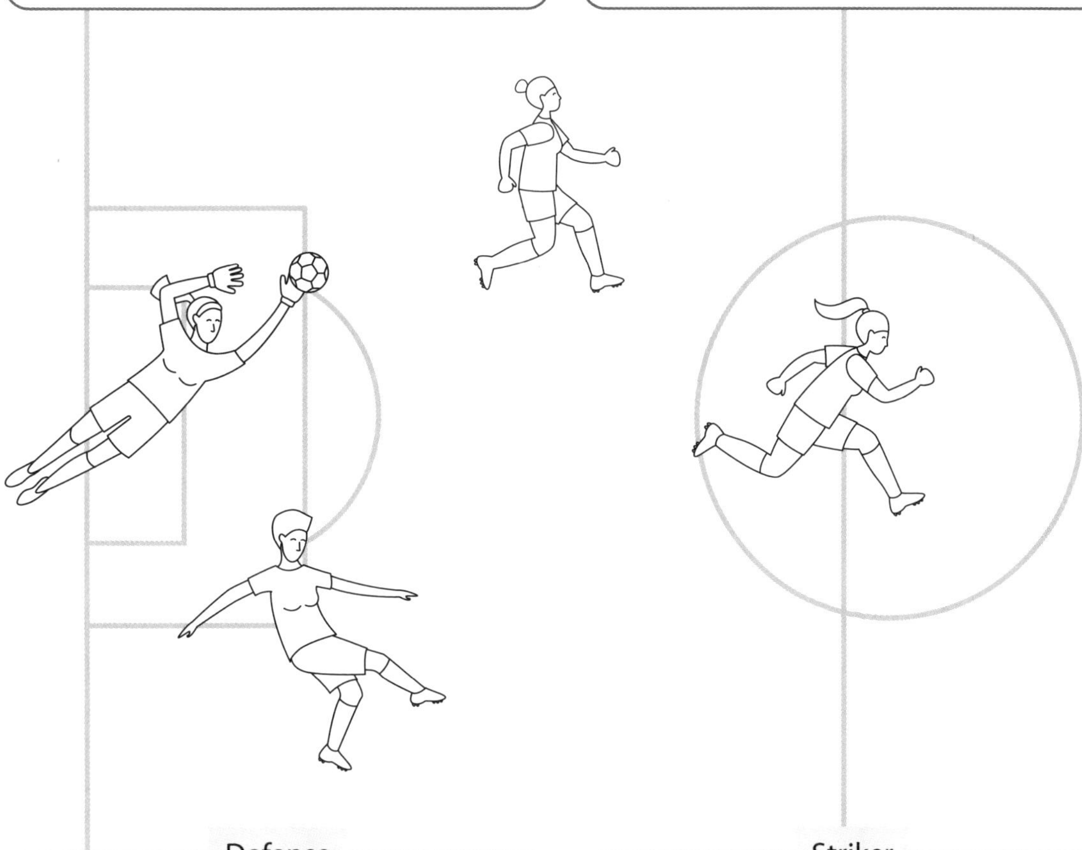

Defense

When facing setbacks, what can you do to protect your progress?

Striker

What actions can you take to pursue your goals?

Who I Am, Who I Want to Be: Part 2

Therapeutic Rationale

This activity builds on the self-reflective work of *Who I Am, Who I Want to Be: Part 1* (see page 155) by helping kids move from insight to behavior change. From an ACT perspective, it supports values-based committed action by translating hopes into realistic, meaningful behaviors.

Goals

- Translate identity-based goals into values-aligned actions
- Break down long-term growth into manageable, purposeful steps

Materials

- *Who I Am, Who I Want to Be* worksheet (completed)
- Writing utensil

Instructions

1. Have the client revisit their completed *Who I Am, Who I Want to Be* worksheet from part 1. Invite them to look at both sections and ask if there's anything they would like to add, change, or explain differently on the worksheet.
2. Direct them to focus on the "Who I Want to Be" section and ask, "What parts of that person already live in you now?" Have the client circle all the qualities that feel true, even in small ways (e.g., kind, brave, good listener, patient).
3. Next, ask, "What would it look like to *act* more like that person today?" Help them name two to three small, realistic actions connected to those qualities. For example, if they want to be someone who is brave even in the face of fear, they might raise their hand in class more often. Write these actions down on the worksheet.
4. Break each action down even further by identifying the concrete steps the client could take to work toward becoming that person (e.g., "During math class tomorrow, I will notice when I have an idea and raise my hand once"). Write these details on the worksheet.
5. Discuss how the person they are today does not need to stand in the way of the person they are becoming. With that in mind, have the client identify some potential challenges that might get in the way of their actions (e.g., "I might worry that I'll get the answer wrong and keep my hand down"). Then help them develop a specific plan for how they will respond if that happens (e.g., "I will remind myself that being brave means trying, not being right").

Remote Control Life

Therapeutic Rationale

"I'll only feel better when the other person does what I want them to do!" Most child therapists have heard their clients say those exact words countless times. Of course, life would be easier if everyone did exactly what we wanted, but the truth is, the only person we can control is ourselves. This exercise helps kids internalize that concept in a playful way.

Goals

- Illustrate that we can only control ourselves
- Promote acceptance of what is out of our control to support committed action

Materials

- Two remote control cars
- Safe space to set up a driving course

Instructions

1. Ask your client if they would like to spend a few minutes playing together with some remote control cars.
2. Then set up a simple course and have a race. It can be helpful to let your client win the first race, although this is optional.
3. After the first race, tell your client that you want a rematch. Once the rematch starts, cheat on purpose by blocking their car, bumping into it, or otherwise interfering. Do not go over the top and upset them too much—the goal is for them to be annoyed.
4. Pause the activity and ask why they are frustrated. When they share their feelings, apologize and note that it can feel really yucky when other people do things that we don't want them to do. Then have another race, and this time, play fairly. Spend a few minutes enjoying the cars together.
5. While continuing to play, ask them to recall another time when they were upset because someone acted in a way that they did not want. Have them take you through it. What was so distressing for them? What did they want the other person to do (or not do)?
6. Next, invite them to try using their remote to "control" your car. Let them notice that no matter how hard they try, it doesn't respond to their remote.
7. Use this to highlight the key lesson: Just like these cars, the only person they can control is themselves. Explore how it feels to realize this, and brainstorm how they can keep this in mind the next time someone else's actions feel frustrating.

Science Experiment

Therapeutic Rationale

Kids often struggle to see the connection between engaging in committed action and feeling better. They'll ask us, "How will *that* do anything?" or "What does *that* have to do with how I'm feeling?" Being the well-intended mad scientists that we are, we will typically suggest a simple experiment. Once the child performs the experiment, they will be able to glean the results for themselves.

Goals

- Facilitate meaningful committed action
- Connect the impact of committed action on overall mental health, wellness, and mood

Materials

- None

Instructions

1. Propose a "bet" with your client. You'll bet that if they follow through with at least one meaningful goal or action consistently, they will likely feel at least a little bit better. Decide together on a motivating reward if they "win" the bet (e.g., extra game time, piece of candy).
2. Have your client choose one goal or meaningful action they've identified in previous activities. Using SMART goal principles, work with them to create a step-by-step plan for completing this goal. Assign the first step (or steps) as homework.
3. Check in with them each week to review their progress, discuss how they are feeling, and point out any changes in their mood or overall well-being as they engage in committed action. Identify any support they may need to continue moving toward their goal.
4. Once they have accomplished the goal, celebrate their effort. Affirm both their choice to try something to feel better and the results they achieved.
5. Process the experience together: Did it impact their life in positive or negative ways? How did it impact their mood? What did they learn about themselves from engaging in this action? Do they think it was helpful or unhelpful to try this? How can they move forward with another meaningful action?
6. Finally, check the outcome of the bet. Whether they "won" or "lost," give them the agreed-upon reward as recognition of their hard work.

Five-Minute Rule

Therapeutic Rationale

One of the biggest barriers to committed action is feeling overwhelmed by how *much* there is to do. The "five-minute rule" offers a practical way to overcome this inertia and avoidance. Based on the concepts of behavioral activation and micro-commitments, it reminds kids that small steps still move them forward. If they can complete a task in five minutes or less, they can and should do it now. If a task feels bigger or harder, they can commit to *just five minutes* of effort and see where it goes. This builds momentum and confidence while aligning their actions with values.

Goals

- Reduce avoidance and procrastination by lowering the barrier to action
- Break down larger tasks into manageable steps

Materials

- Blank paper
- Writing utensil
- Stopwatch or timer (optional)

Instructions

1. Ask your client to think about the small tasks that they often delay, avoid, or ignore. Many of these tasks can be completed quickly—in five minutes or less—but they still put them off. Explain that doing even one of these small tasks can create a sense of accomplishment and reduce mental clutter, making it easier to take other actions later.
2. Invite your client to write down a list of tasks they need to complete today or this week. Then have them go through the list and circle the ones that can be done in five minutes or less.
3. If the client struggles to come up with anything, here are some examples you can offer them:
    - Texting a friend back
    - Packing their backpack
    - Writing down their homework
    - Tidying part of their room
    - Taking a few deep breaths
    - Drinking a glass of water
    - Setting out clothes for tomorrow
4. Ask what is one thing they can do now, in the next five minutes, to take a small step toward their goals—and have them do it! You can set a timer for added effect.
5. Encourage them to continue this process throughout the week to build momentum. Whenever they encounter a task they can do in under five minutes, have them commit to doing it right then and there!

Take Your Thoughts to Court

Therapeutic Rationale

Many kids struggle with poor self-concept, insecure attachment, and low self-efficacy. As therapists, we act as temporary surrogate attachment figures, helping kids stand up to their biggest bullies: themselves. This exercise uses a courtroom metaphor that provides kids with a humorous way to challenge their own unhelpful thoughts. It is most effective when a child shares a thought that is shaped by emotional reasoning. By treating their thought as a "case" in court, clients can examine evidence, test the validity of their beliefs, and strengthen their sense of self.

Goals

- Improve psychological flexibility via humor
- Disrupt the cycle of self-defeating thoughts

Materials

- Blank paper
- Writing utensil

Instructions

1. Introduce the activity: "Sometimes, we assume that every single thought our brain throws at us is true. That's exhausting! What if we got better at sorting out the true stuff from the untrue stuff?" Explain that today they will be taking their thought to court to see if it holds up under scrutiny.
2. Introduce the roles of the courtroom:
   a. **Prosecutor:** Presents evidence that the thought is *true*
   b. **Defense counsel:** Presents counterevidence to show that the thought is *false*
   c. **Jury:** Weighs the evidence and decides whether the thought is true
   d. **Judge:** Guides the process and reads the verdict
3. Remind them that evidence means evidence—not a feeling, not a fear, not a hunch. If it wouldn't hold up in a court of law, then it isn't going to hold up in this courtroom either.
4. Have your client assemble their jury by selecting supportive people (real or imagined) who stand up for them. This could include caregivers, teachers, friends, or fictional characters. Explain that in life, supportive people act like a jury by helping us weigh evidence fairly. If you believe the client would benefit from a more concrete visual, have them draw and label their jury box and members.
5. Once the jury is assembled, identify a thought to put on trial. It could be "Nobody likes me," "I'm unworthy of love," or "I'm annoying."

6. Have your client act as the prosecutor first. Ask them to gather evidence that this thought is true and present it to the jury. This may seem counterintuitive, but it is critical to the exercise. It is very difficult to imagine telling friends, loved ones, or heroes that you are a terrible person. Imagine telling Mister Rogers that you don't deserve to be loved—he obviously wouldn't accept that. The point is to give the client a safe space to practice challenging unhelpful beliefs.
7. Next, ask them to act as the defense counsel. Have them gather evidence that this thought is false and present it to the jury.
8. Finally, have them take on the role of the judge who is about to make a ruling. Invite the client to consider the "testimony" presented the court. What do they imagine the jury has decided? Will it find that the thought is true or untrue? What might be a more balanced or adaptive thought?
9. If the jury finds that the thought is true, repeat the exercise, but this time determining whether it is a helpful or unhelpful thought. Ultimately, most distressing thoughts are untrue, unhelpful, or both, so no matter what, you can help the client to restructure their beliefs.

Bricks in the Wall

Therapeutic Rationale

People are all different, but heartache, a fear of the future, and a dislike for change are all near-universal human experiences. One common experience is feeling overwhelmed. Who hasn't been paralyzed by a challenge that seems too big to tackle? This exercise is designed to help kids acknowledge those feelings, calm them, and identify strategies to overcome them.

Goals

- Make perceived obstacles feel less overwhelming
- Provide a metaphorical reframing of "insurmountable" obstacles

Materials

- *Brick Wall* template
- Writing utensil

Instructions

1. Ask your client to share one of their goals that feels overwhelming or insurmountable.
2. Introduce the brick wall metaphor: In these situations, it can feel as though we are standing in front of a massive brick wall. No matter how much we try to climb it, go around it, or knock it down, we remain stuck behind it. Ask the client to reflect on what it feels like for them when this happens.
3. Explain that one of the best ways to tackle the wall is to knock it down one brick at a time. Each brick represents a barrier—something that is blocking progress toward their goal.
4. Share the *Brick Wall* template and have the client write their goal on the other side of the wall. Then work together to identify and label the bricks that are acting as barriers to that goal. For example, if a client's goal is to win the science fair, potential barriers may include:
    - Not knowing how to design the experiment
    - Difficulty managing time between schoolwork and the project
    - Fear of presenting in front of the judges
5. Once all bricks are fully labeled, help the client identify which bricks seem the most breakable. Come up with a plan to mitigate, change, or overcome those specific barriers. Continuing with the science fair example, this might include the following:
    - Asking a teacher for guidance on the design
    - Setting up mini deadlines for each step of the project
    - Practicing the presentation in front of family or friends
6. Remind your client that they do not need to remove every single brick to knock down the wall. Often, removing enough of the load-bearing bricks will bring the wall down.

Brick Wall Template

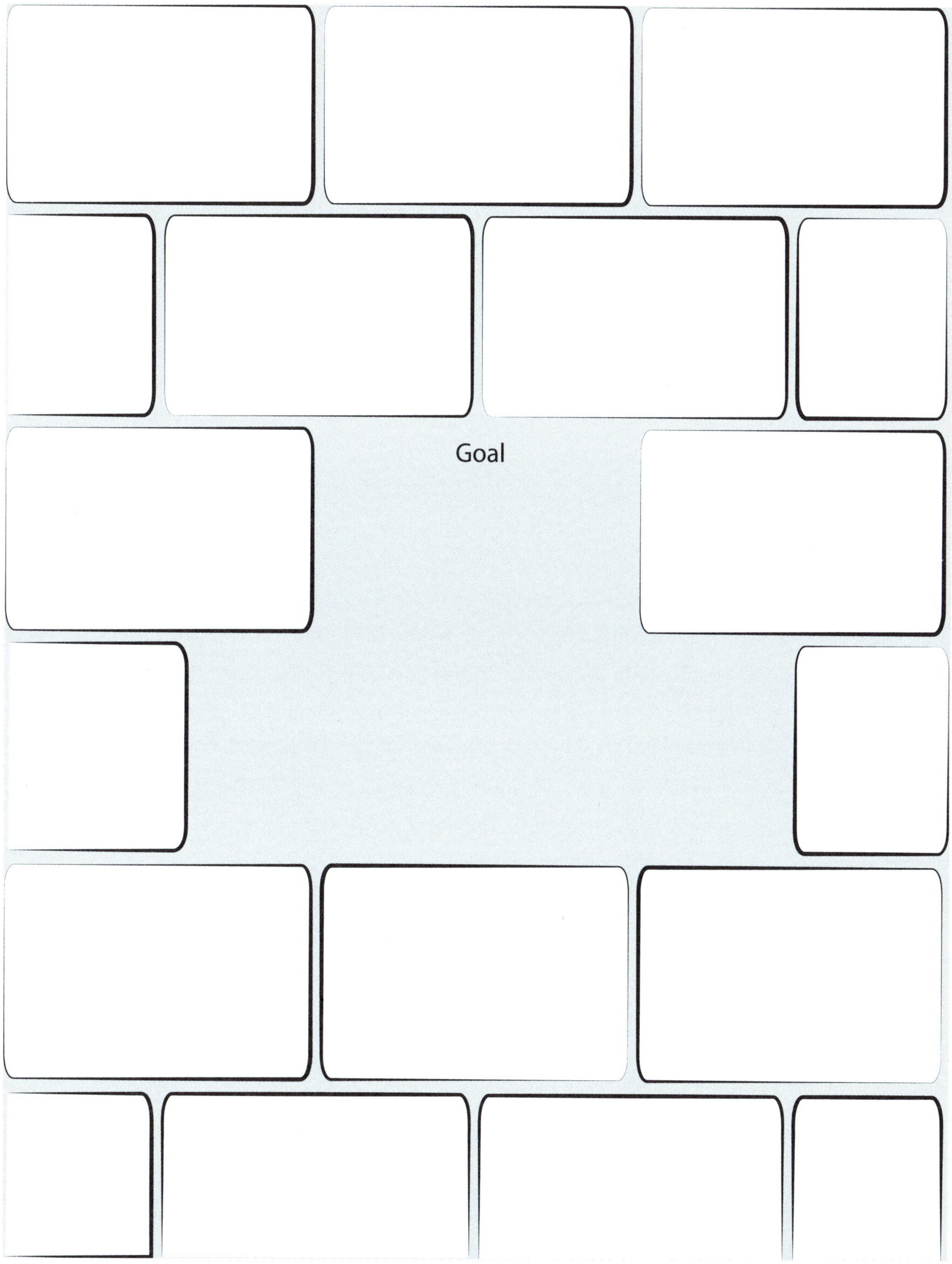

Marathon Goals

Therapeutic Rationale

Running a marathon is an exercise in pacing and perspective. At 26.2 miles, even trained runners can feel overwhelmed if they focus on the entire course. Instead, they have to think about it in bite-sized pieces: "I've done the first five miles! I can do that again." "Oh wow, already at 13.1 miles! That wasn't easy, but I can do that again, and now I'm over the 50 percent mark." Life works much the same way. We don't need to tackle everything all at once; we can take a step or two forward toward the finish line. Using our available resources, we can train up to our goal—one mile, one task, one step at a time. This activity draws on the marathon metaphor by applying a strengths-based approach to goal setting rather than a traditional fear hierarchy.

Goals

- Reframe fears and anxieties
- Increase psychological flexibility and defuse from anxiety

Materials

- *Marathon Goals* worksheet
- Writing utensil

Instructions

1. Start by clarifying your client's ultimate goal—something they want to accomplish but don't feel capable of achieving. Write that goal on the *Marathon Goals* worksheet. Remind your client that the goal is not to complete this all at once, just like a runner doesn't run 26.2 miles in a single step.
2. Work together to break the goal into incremental "courage steps." For example, if the goal is to give a speech in front of a large crowd, the first step may be to imagine giving the speech. The second step may be practicing alone in front of the mirror. Emphasize that it's better to have too many steps than to have too few.
3. For each "courage step," write down the personal values it aligns with, the elements of the hexaflex it corresponds with, and how willing the client is currently to be courageous enough to perform that step. (Review the hexaflex with the client if needed.) Remind your client that courage isn't the absence of fear. It is being afraid and doing it anyway.
4. Have your client gradually progress through the plan. Before they complete each "courage step," check in: What internal and external resources do they need to "run that part of the race"? What will increase their willingness to courageously complete the task?
5. Work through the plan, adjusting it as necessary. Part of the goal is to help the client defuse from unhelpful thoughts and feelings. Instead of thinking "I can't do it because it is too scary," they must think, "It was scary, and I was still able to do it because I am awesome." Remind your client that "scary" does not mean "bad"—it often signals that the task is important to them.

Marathon Goals Worksheet

Use this worksheet to break down your goal into smaller "courage steps." For each step, record what personal values it connects to, what part of the hexaflex it uses, and how willing you are to be courageous (0 = not willing, 10 = very willing).

Goal: ____

Courage Step	Personal Value	Hexaflex Focus	Willingness to be Courageous (0–10)

Rowboat

Therapeutic Rationale

This activity helps kids visualize their life journey as a rowing trip: They sometimes take steady strokes forward, while other times it can feel like they are spinning in circles. It normalizes moments of stuckness, confusion, or exhaustion while encouraging them to pause, reorient, and recommit to their goals.

Goals

- Promote self-awareness when progress feels stuck or cyclical
- Practice flexible problem-solving and intentional recommitment

Materials

- *Rowboat* template
- Writing utensil
- Crayons, markers, or colored pencils (optional)

Instructions

1. Introduce the *Rowboat* template and ask the client to imagine that they are in this boat, rowing toward their goals. They can draw themselves in the boat if they would like.
2. Have the client draw or write in obstacles in the water that keep them spinning in circles (i.e., prevent them from reaching this goal)—for example, waves, whirlpools, storms, floating logs, or even sea monsters.
3. If the client struggles to identify obstacles, offer the following prompts:
   a. "What's something that has made you feel stuck?"
   b. "When was a time you were working hard but didn't feel like you were making any progress or going anywhere?"
4. Explain that even the strongest rowers sometimes drift off course or get tired, so they need to pause and reorient from time to time ask themselves the following questions:
   a. "What direction am I rowing in right now?"
   b. "Is it toward a value and goal? Why or why not?"
   c. "What is making it hard to go in the right direction or to continue on?"
   d. "If I keep rowing in this direction, where will I end up?"
5. To help the client "steer" their boat in a new direction, help them make a new rowing plan. Have the client complete the following prompts on the bottom of the template:
   a. My anchor value is _________.
   b. A small action I can take today to row in that direction is ___________.
   c. If I start rowing in circles, I can do this to help me stay on track: ____________.
   d. Tools or people who help me stay on track are ____________.

Rowboat Template

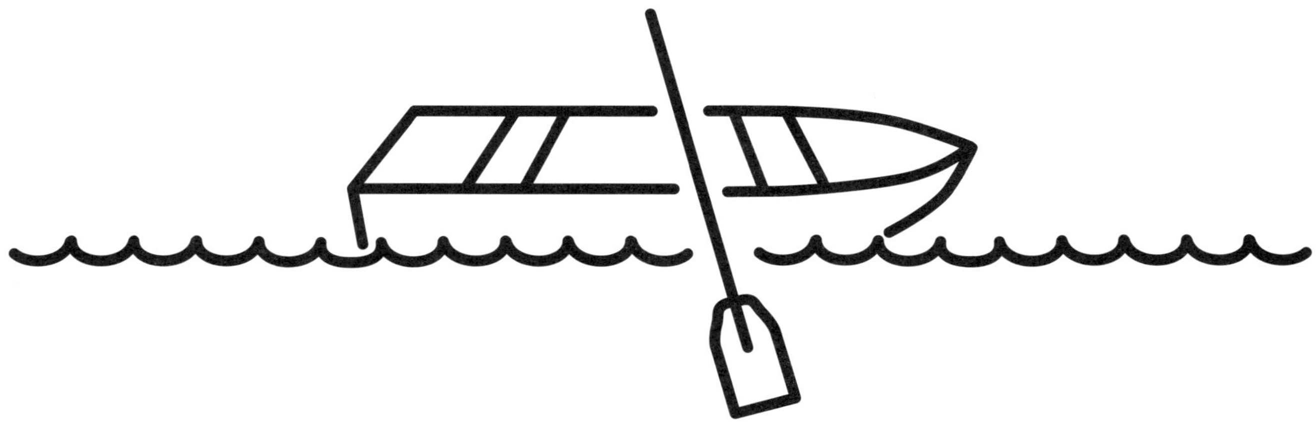

My anchor value is ______________________________.

A small action I can take today to row in that direction is ______________________________

______________________________.

If I start rowing in circles, I can do this to help me stay on track: ______________________________.

____

Tools or people who help me stay on track are ______________________________

______________________________.

Web of Why

Therapeutic Rationale

Committed action is most sustainable when it is grounded it in our "why." When we lose sight of why we're making hard choices or taking uncomfortable steps, we can feel disconnected, frustrated, or lost. This activity helps kids visualize their daily actions and values as interconnected threads, all woven together into a larger spiderweb of a meaningful life. Each thread—choice, effort, setback, success—is part of that web that holds and supports them.

Goals

- Strengthen motivation by connecting actions to deeply held values
- Increase awareness of how small actions contribute to a larger whole

Materials

- *Spiderweb* template
- Writing utensil
- Crayons, markers, or colored pencils

Instructions

1. Introduce the *Spiderweb* template and have the client write in their goals and values in the center of the web. (These should have been identified in previous activities.)
2. In each concentric circle radiating out from the center of the web, have them write down supports that move them toward those values and goals. This might include family members or friends, hobbies, therapy, personal strengths, skills, or self-care practices. Encourage them to think broadly.
3. Next, focus on the lines that connect the circles to the center. Along each line, have them answer these "why" questions:
    a. "Why does this matter to you?
    b. "Why do you keep working toward this goal or value?"
    c. "What sometimes holds me back, and what can you do to keep going?"
4. Point out that if one thread breaks or frays, the whole web doesn't collapse. The web has many strong points holding it together, and new threads can be rebuilt or added as needed.
5. Finally, ask the client to draw in new lines to the web representing small, concrete steps they can take to keep moving forward toward their goals.

Spiderweb Template

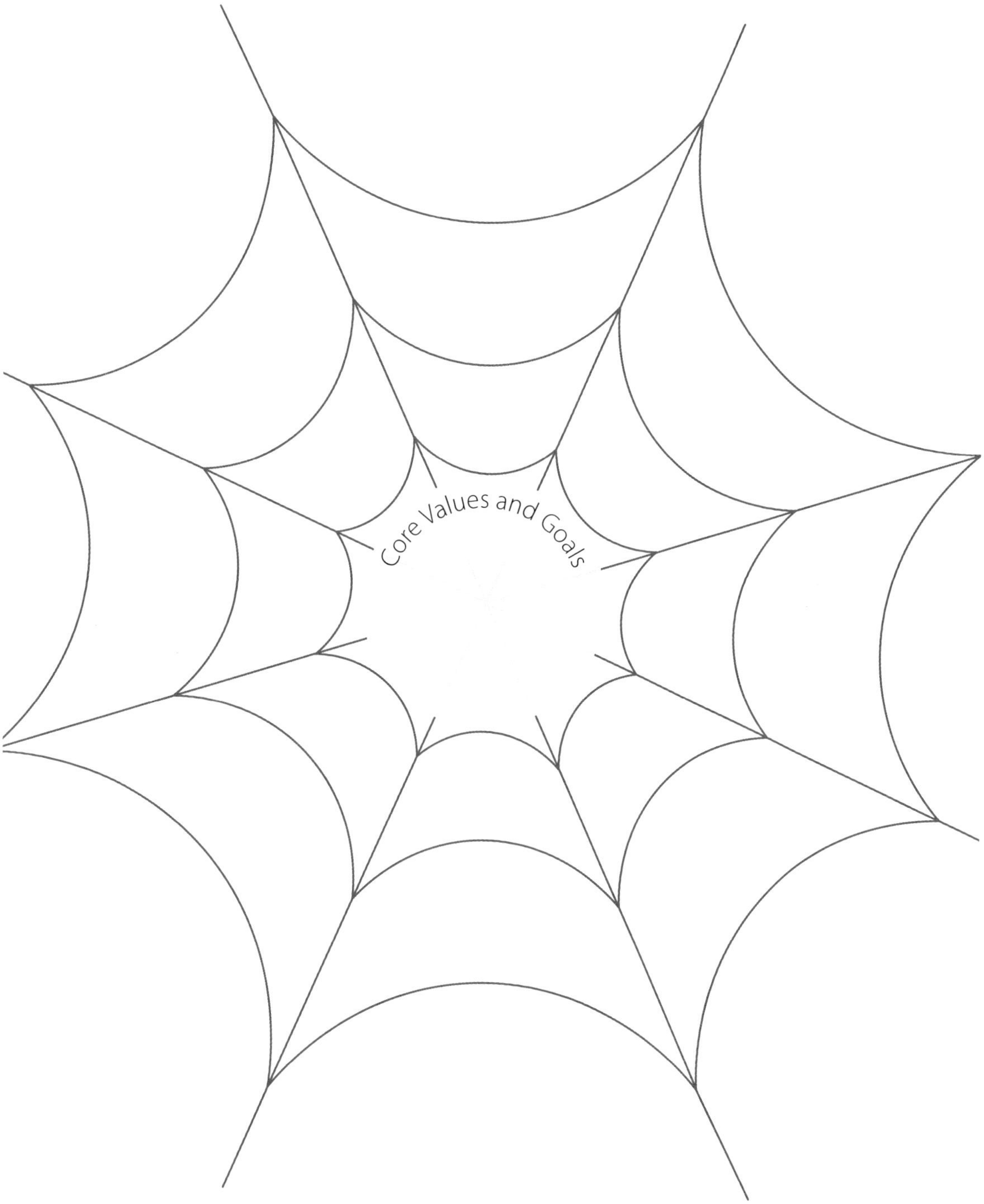

Quicksand

Therapeutic Rationale

When we are caught in distressing thoughts or emotions, our natural response is often to fight, escape, or push harder. However, just like struggling in quicksand, the more we resist, the more stuck we become. This activity uses the quicksand metaphor to help kids recognize how resistance can make distress worse, whereas slowing down, accepting the situation, and taking values-based steps forward can help them escape the quicksand rather than continuing to sink deeper.

Goals

- Increase awareness of emotional and behavioral avoidance
- Build insight into how resistance can backfire
- Encourage taking small concrete steps in the direction of values

Materials

- Blank paper
- Writing utensil
- Computer with speakers (optional)

Instructions

1. Introduce the metaphor: "Imagine you are stuck in quicksand. What's your first instinct?" Pause to allow the client to answer, then explain, "Most people think they need to push the sand away, fight against it, or kick hard to climb out really fast. But the more you fight, the deeper you sink."
2. Then explain, "What actually helps in quicksand is slowing down, remaining calm, spreading out your weight, and making slow, intentional movements."
3. You can also show a video of someone escaping quicksand so the client can visualize this more easily.
4. Connect the metaphor to real life: "Life can feel like quicksand at times. These are the moments we feel trapped, overwhelmed, or stuck. Often, our first instinct is to run, escape, or ignore the problem—but just like with quicksand, those reactions make us sink deeper."
5. Ask the client to reflect on a recent "quicksand" moment in their life and have them briefly describe it. What did they do in that moment? Guide them to identify which of the following strategies they used:
    a. Fought against it
    b. Ran away (mentally or in real life)
    c. Froze or shut down

d. Paused, made a plan, and took a step toward their values
e. Used another strategy

6. Explain that the first step in getting out of quicksand (or any sticky situation) is to pause, notice, and accept the situation. Acceptance doesn't mean that the situation is easy or that they like it, but it prevents them from sinking further. Have the client list a few strategies that help them slow down and practice acceptance (e.g., taking deep breaths, reminding themselves that thoughts and feelings are temporary).
7. The next step is to shift to planning: "Now that you've paused and accepted the situation, you can think about where you want to go. Based on the sticky situation you described, what would have been a good plan of action?" For example, if they skipped a birthday party for a new friend because they were afraid they wouldn't know anyone, a good plan might have been to decide to attend for at least 10 minutes or to identify one person they could talk to in advance.
8. Finally, make a plan for the future: "Next time a similar situation happens, what are one or two things you could do right away to take the first step?" Encourage the client to brainstorm small actions they could try to make them less likely to "sink" next time.

Mindful Moments of Joy

Therapeutic Rationale

We often imagine that change occurs through big, dramatic actions. While this can happen occasionally, lasting change usually occurs via evolution, not revolution—in other words, through small, intentional steps. Making time to experience joy is one of those small steps. Even though moments of joy are temporary, they help nurture our hearts and minds and make it easier to cope with challenges. This activity helps kids do just that.

Goals

- Implement intentional joyful moments in daily life
- Engage in meaningful actions that nurture emotional and mental well-being

Materials

- Blank paper and writing utensil (optional)

Instructions

1. Ask your client to remember the last time they intentionally created a moment of joy—not a moment that happened by accident, but something that they planned for. How often do they intentionally create such moments on a regular basis?
2. Explore the importance of joy, explaining that it nurtures our heart and soul. Ask the client to reflect on what part of them could use some nurturing and what that might look like. These moments can be small, like eating a favorite food or reading a favorite book, or larger, like spending the day doing something special. Brainstorm ideas with your client.
3. How does thinking about these joyful moments make the client feel in the here and now? What do they feel in their body as you have this conversation? Are any emotions coming up? What might those feelings be trying to tell them about what they need or enjoy?
4. Together, create a plan to engage in moments of joy over the coming month. This might involve trying a new hobby or planning a special outing with family or friends. Encourage concrete actions! Assign these moments of joy for homework, and then process the experience in future sessions.
5. If helpful, write these ideas down so the client can remember them outside of session.

Coping Chef

Therapeutic Rationale

When life serves up big emotions, tough situations, or overwhelming thoughts, we need the right coping "ingredients" to support ourselves. In ACT, mindfulness helps us notice what's happening *without judgment*, while committed action involves *choosing responses* that align with our values. This activity invites kids to create their own personalized "menu" of coping strategies they can reach for when things get hard. Just like a chef chooses ingredients to match a recipe and taste, kids will learn to mindfully choose which skill best fits what they need at the moment.

Goals

- Mindfully reflect on the most effective coping tools
- Increase awareness of emotional needs and how to respond to them

Materials

- *Coping Skills Menu* template
- Writing utensil
- Paper chef hats and crayons, markers, or colored pencils (optional)

Instructions

1. Introduce the activity: "When big emotions show up, we need coping skills that match what we're dealing with. Just like a chef chooses different foods for different recipes, we can choose different coping skills depending on how intense things feel."
2. Walk the client through the *Coping Skills Menu* template, and work with the client to create their own personalized menu. Explain that you are going to sort coping skills based on *how much* they help as well as *when* they work best:
    a. **Appetizers:** Quick coping skills that help a little or take the edge off
    b. **Main course:** Stronger coping skills that help a lot, especially when an "appetizer" didn't "fill them up"
    c. **Dessert:** Coping skills that help the client settle, recover, and reground
    d. **Chef's special:** Fun or situation-specific skills that work well only in certain places or times (e.g., petting a dog might help at home but not during class).
3. **Optional:** Decorate chef's hats to help make the activity more fun and help the client feel ownership over their coping tools.

Coping Skills Menu Template

MENU

Appetizers

Main Course

Desserts

Chef's Special!

Progress Over Perfection

Therapeutic Rationale

Committed action isn't about achieving perfect outcomes—it's about choosing to move toward our values with flexibility, courage, and persistence. This activity supports kids in shifting away from perfectionism and performance-based thinking and toward effort-based self-reflection. Kids often hold themselves to rigid standards, which can lead to avoidance, shame, or burnout when they fall short. By helping them notice and appreciate the progress they are making—even in small or imperfect steps—we strengthen their ability to stay on a values-aligned path no matter the outcome.

Goals

- Reinforce values-based action as more important than "perfect" performance
- Normalize mistakes, setbacks, and challenges as part of growth
- Encourage self-compassion and reflection

Materials

- *Progress Over Perfection* worksheet
- Writing utensil

Instructions

1. Begin by exploring the client's current understanding of perfectionism: "What does being perfect mean to you?" and "Do you ever feel like things, or you yourself, need to be exactly right?"
2. Use this discussion to normalize the experience of perfectionistic thinking and introduce the idea that focusing on progress and values (rather than perfect outcomes) can reduce pressure and stress: "Sometimes we get stuck thinking that we have to do something perfectly for it to matter. But growth usually happens through small steps, stumbles, mistakes, and trying again. When we focus on progress, we notice how far we've come—not just how far we have to go."
3. Introduce the *Progress Over Perfection* worksheet, and invite the client to reflect on a specific action they took over the past week that moved them toward a value they care about. Stress that even "small" or "imperfect" actions count.
4. As they work through the questions, help them notice where perfectionistic thinking shows up (e.g., "It didn't go well enough," "I should have done more"). Redirect their attention to the *process* over the product and the *effort* over the outcome by asking, "What value were you honoring by simply showing up and trying?"

5. After completing the worksheet, guide the client to mindfully notice and appreciate their effort with some reflection prompts:
    a. "What do you feel proud of?"
    b. "How could you celebrate this small step?"
    c. "How can you continue to remind yourself that even small progress counts?"
6. Invite the client to keep the worksheet in a folder or journal to track their progress over time.
7. **Optional:** Ask the client to complete the activity between sessions (daily or at a pace that feels right) to review their progress next session.

Progress Over Perfection Worksheet

What is one thing you did this week that moved you toward a value you care about? Remember that big or small, every step forward counts.

____

____

Did it go exactly how you wanted it to? Why or why not?

____

____

What helped you keep going even when it was hard or less than perfect? Did you use a coping skill or practice self-care? Did you ask for help? Did you practice being kind to yourself?

____

____

What are you proud of yourself for in this situation?

____

____

What is one small step you could take next to keep moving forward?

____

____

Taking Care of Who You Will Be Tomorrow

Therapeutic Rationale

"Self-care" is a phrase that's everywhere, and while it's certainly an important part of wellness, it can be tricky because pretty much anything can be done in the name of self-care. Eating a whole bag of candy in one sitting? Self-care! Staying up super late to play video games? Self-care! Skipping chores because it feels hard? Self-care! In truth, self-care is about taking care of who we will be tomorrow. It asks us to pause and consider the long-term impact of our choices. Tomorrow, will we be grateful that we skipped our homework and stayed up playing video games? Or will we feel more stressed? The answer will probably be different every time, and that's okay. This activity helps kids move beyond an "anything goes" mentality regarding self-care and toward more intentional, values-aligned actions.

Goals

- Differentiate between self-care and self-indulgence
- Promote intentional and meaningful self-care actions

Materials

- None

Instructions

1. Introduce the idea that self-care is about taking care of the version of ourselves that will exist *tomorrow*. It isn't just about doing what feels good in the moment, but thinking ahead and considering how we will feel when we wake up tomorrow.
2. Ask your client to consider a time when they performed "self-care" that wound up making things harder the next day, as well as a time when they engaged in self-care that did help them feel better the next day. What was the difference between the two experiences?
3. Work with the client to pause and consider what "tomorrow them" needs right now. What can they do today that their future self will be thankful for? Work together to identify one or two realistic actions they can take that would support their future self.

Pre-negotiating Reasons *Not* to Do Something

Therapeutic Rationale

Stand-up comedian Mitch Hedberg once said, "I write jokes for a living, I sit at my hotel at night, I think of something that's funny, then I go get a pen and I write it down. Or if the pen is too far away, I have to convince myself that what I thought of ain't funny." This quote demonstrates a universal truth: When a goal feels too challenging or uncomfortable, we often work to convince ourselves that we didn't really want it anyway. It's easier to pretend that we're okay with not trying because trying (especially trying and failing) is just too scary. This exercise is designed to help kids move beyond that fear.

Goals

- Build resilience and perseverance
- Promote psychological flexibility
- Minimize all-or-nothing thinking

Materials

- None

Instructions

1. When your client expresses reluctance to pursue a desired path, approach it with curiosity. Why are they rethinking their goals? What feels scary or difficult about the potential path forward?
2. Explain that comfort and growth rarely coexist. It is very difficult to grow while remaining comfortable the entire time. However, when something feels challenging, we start coming up with reasons to stay in our comfort zone. This is normal, but it stops us from reaching our goals.
3. Ask your client to notice what thoughts and feelings come up when they think about the task or goal they are avoiding. What is their heart telling them? How is their brain trying to protect them from potential failure?
4. Gently challenge them to consider the source of their hesitation: Is their second-guessing coming from their values, or is it coming from a place of fear? Regardless of their answer, help them name and express what they are thinking and feeling.
5. Guide your client through a brief mindfulness or grounding exercise to calm their body before you move on to the next step of the activity.
6. Collaborate with them to identify a committed action that aligns with their values, not fear. Remind them that these steps don't have to be perfect—they just need to move them forward.
7. To close, summarize this process and remind your client of the four steps for handling discomfort: (1) notice what they are feeling and thinking, (2) name and express it verbally, (3) calm the body using mindfulness or grounding, and (4) take a step toward committed action based on values, not fear.

Hobby Hunter

Therapeutic Rationale

This activity encourages kids to explore their personal interests with curiosity and intentionality rather than pressure or performance. When kids pursue their hobbies in a mindful way, it helps build joy, agency, and values-driven action, especially when motivation is low or perfectionism takes over. This activity helps them notice what sparks their interest, identify manageable steps forward, and practice being present as they explore those sparks.

Goals

- Reconnect with interests, passions, and curiosity
- Foster mindfulness by slowing down and staying present during exploration

Materials

- Blank paper
- Writing utensil
- Stopwatch or timer

Instructions

1. Ask the client to think about things they love doing, things they have always been curious about, or things they enjoy learning about.
2. Set a timer for two minutes and ask the client to make a list of anything that comes to mind. There are no "right" or "wrong" answers. Anything that sparks interest can be included, whether it's a hobby they currently do, an activity they are passionate about, or something they have always wanted to try.
3. Once the list is complete, have them go back and underline the items that stand out most. Which ones call to them?
4. Now have the client look at the underlined items and have them circle the ones that they want to take meaningful steps toward pursuing.
5. Then encourage the client to spend a few minutes each day engaging with the activities or interests they underlined. For example: research or learn more about that hobby (e.g., watch videos, read articles); try out a version of the hobby; journal about what they liked or noticed while exploring the hobby; draw, doodle, or talk about the hobby.
6. As the client explores their hobby over the next week, encourage them to practice being present. Notice what thoughts or feelings show up—whether it's excitement, nervousness, boredom, or frustration—and let them pass like clouds. Then return their attention to the moment.
7. At the next session, ask the client to reflect on the experience. What hobby or idea did they connect with the most? How did it feel to explore something without pressure or judgment? What did they learn about themselves in the process?

Growth Over Time

Therapeutic Rationale

Change doesn't always look like big, visible progress. Sometimes we grow quietly, slowly, or beneath the surface. Just like plants, we may need rest, nourishment, or a change in conditions before we bloom again. This reflection activity encourages kids to mindfully notice how far they've come, even when growth feels invisible. It also normalizes the need for rest and support, reminding kids that slow seasons are still part of the growth process.

Goals

- Reflect on personal growth and celebrate small progress
- Increase awareness of internal and external needs (e.g., rest, support, space)

Materials

- Blank paper
- Writing utensil

Instructions

1. For this activity, invite the client to draw, journal, or talk through the following reflection questions.
2. Ask the client to look back and consider how far they've come:
    a. "What is something you can do now that you couldn't do before?"
    b. "What challenges did you face this year, month, or week?"
    c. "What's one small step you took toward something that matters to you?"
3. Next, normalize slow periods when growth pauses:
    a. "Have there been times when you felt "stuck" or like you weren't growing?"
    b. "What do you think they you doing during that time (e.g., resting, surviving, gathering, strength, planning)?"
    c. "What would you say to a plant that hasn't grown yet? Would you give it kindness or criticism?"
4. Help the client identify what supports and nourishes them, allowing them to flourish:
    a. "What helps you grow even when growth is hard?"
    b. "What kind of "water" or "sunlight" do you need more of right now?"
    c. "Who or what helps you feel more like yourself again?"
5. Finally, ask what next steps they can take to keep moving forward:
    a. "What's one way you can gently support your own growth this week?"
    b. "What's something you want to *notice* more, like a tiny leaf growing or a quiet moment of courage?"

Acknowledgments

This book was created by therapists, for therapists, to try to make ACT more accessible to children and adolescents. We would like to express our deep gratitude to PESI for being just as passionate about supporting clinicians as we are. Specific thanks to Roseanne Cheng for believing in this project from the start.

We would also like to recognize all the helpers out there who picked up this book with the sole intention of helping someone else. We would also like to acknowledge those who guided us along our own journey, including Ryan Zoltowski, the Heydt family, Dr. Dina del Amo, Dr. Erin Adamitis, James Wrona, Dr. Matt Snyder, Chase Utley, and the Ercolani family.

About the Authors

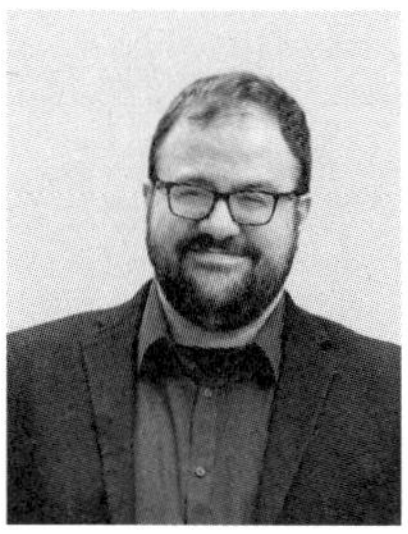

Matt Ercolani, MS, LPC, NCC, is a licensed professional counselor based in Pennsylvania. He has worked in a variety of settings throughout his career, including partial hospitalization, intensive outpatient, substance use rehabilitation, outpatient, and private practice settings. He currently works in a private practice, where he primarily uses ACT and attachment theory in his counseling work with queer and trans youth and their families. Matt is also in demand as a consultant and presenter, having presented throughout the country on topics including working with queer clients, ACT, and mitigating anxiety in educational settings. He is currently completing his doctoral work in counseling and supervision at James Madison University in Virginia.

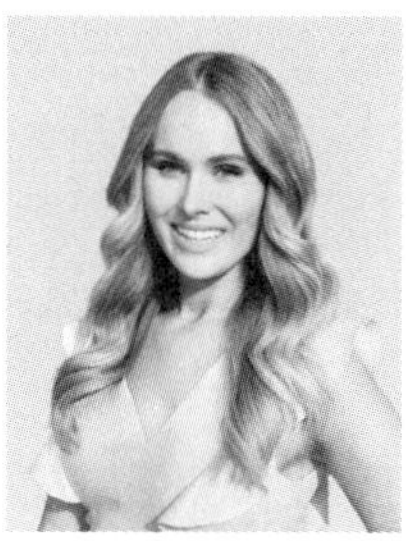

Dr. Emily Heydt, PsyD, is a certified school psychologist and postdoctoral fellow who has extensive experience providing school-based and outpatient mental health services to children, adolescents, young adults, and their families. She earned her doctorate of psychology in school psychology and has focused her career on helping neurodiverse individuals and their families. Dr. Heydt currently specializes in neuro-affirming therapy and evaluations and also provides nationwide presentations focused on supporting children and teens through a neuro-affirming and ACT-based lens.